GETTING MY BOUNCE BACK

How I Got Fit, Healthier, and Happier (And You Can, Too)

CAROLEE BELKIN WALKER

Wellness blogger and freelance writer for the *Washington Post,*
Huffington Post, and *Thrive Global* contributor

Published by Mango Publishing Group, a division of Mango Media Inc.

Cover and Layout Design: Elina Diaz

For permission requests, please contact the publisher at:

Mango Publishing Group
2850 Douglas Road, 3rd Floor
Coral Gables, FL 33134 USA
info@mango.bz

For special orders, quantity sales, course adoptions and corporate sales, please email the publisher at sales@mango.bz. For trade and wholesale sales, please contact Ingram Publisher Services at customer.service@ingramcontent.com or +1.800.509.4887.

Getting My Bounce Back: How I Got Fit, Healthier, and Happier (And You Can, Too)

Library of Congress Cataloging

ISBN: (print) 978-1-63353-710-1 (ebook) 978-1-63353-711-8
Library of Congress Control Number: 2017964328
BISAC category code: BISAC category code HEA010000 HEALTH & FITNESS / Healthy Living BISAC category code HEA024000 HEALTH & FITNESS / Women's Health

Printed in the United States of America

For my family, I love you all.

Praise

"Exercise and fitness support our life. It makes us strong—physically, emotionally, and psychologically. It keeps our heart pumping. It promises that we will be able to keep at our life's work longer than if we did not move and that we will someday take our children's children's children swimming in the ocean when we are 98. It is a joyful experience and we get to do it. How lucky are we to be able to support our life like this? As Carolee would say: 'You got this.'"

—Sarajean Rudman, from the Foreword

"Carolee Walker's Getting My Bounce Back *is an engaging and inspiring read. Getting fit and training to compete in endurance events is no walk in the park, even for the hardiest among us. There are few books out there that genuinely describe the ups and downs of reinventing yourself at midlife while simultaneously teaching us how we can all do it. In this memoir, Carolee's authentic voice shines through as she describes her personal journey of self-discovery and personal mastery. Carolee's journey is instructive, funny, relatable, and most of all, inspiring."*

—Chris Friesen, PhD, sport & performance neuropsychologist and author of the *High Achievement Handbook series*

"Getting my bounce back are the words every runner needs to hear. Often we are shown images and words that portray an easy connection between starting a fitness journey and reaching the moment where everything is easy (although as an elite runner, I know that it never truly becomes easy, you just get tougher). Most books and publications just show the end result, as if we magically appear at the peak of fitness and ideal look, but Carolee allows us to peek into her inner mind, showing us that there is a journey behind those photos, and a point where a health journey switches over from the 'lose weight mentality' to realizing the joy and light exercise brings us in more valuable and meaningful ways. For anyone who has ever wondered why everyone else made it seem so easy, this book is for you."

—Tina Muir, elite runner and host of the *Running for Real* podcast

CONTENTS

CONTENTS

FOREWORD

Within the philosophy of action theory, there are two prerequisites that can lead to action: desire and belief. If we are hungry and *desire* to be full, and we *believe* a sandwich will satisfy that desire, we will eat the sandwich. But are these truly the prerequisites to *committed* action? What about the case for daily exercise: we *desire* to be at a certain level of physical fitness, and we *believe* that daily exercise will lead us to that level of physical fitness. According to action theory, we should all exercise daily. So why is it that so many people do not act, day after day? Why is it sometimes easy to exercise and sometimes not? What makes us commit? There must be more. Something bigger than us. Something that can lead to *committed* action.

Yes, there is. And it is different for everyone.

It is true that we can commit to exercising before work, or join a fitness club with a goal of going to classes daily, or set our sights on a running goal. We might even achieve those goals, to some extent, and for some amount of time. More than likely, however, once the goal is met, or once we grow bored of trying, we will stop doing what we are doing and go back to simply *desiring* a more fit life that we *believe* can be achieved through fitness goals, but with the bizarre inability to propel ourselves into action. The key word being: *ourselves*.

When asked what really lights you up, you probably do not answer: "Myself." Humans, in general, come equipped with a certain set of values. These are values that they have collected over time and grown into, often passed down to them from their foremothers and forefathers. It is building a house of commitment upon the concrete foundation of one's values that creates the ability to take action: chronic action, habitual action, life-changing action, *committed* action. If we build the house of commitment upon a foundation of "should" or "need" or "ourselves," we might as well have built it upon a pile of sand. We will inevitably tire of ourselves or break the rules we've made for ourselves. A house built on sand will crumble the moment action comes blowing in the wind. Brick by brick, stone by stone, we will be left with nothing but a pile of our own unsatisfied desires, charred by the subtle fire of what we once believed to be the solution, no longer willing or able to act on those beliefs for fear of being burned again.

Burned by *ourselves*.

This is bigger than *ourselves*.

Start by figuring out what in this life is most important to you. Maybe it is family, nature, or loyalty. Maybe it is being creative, fun-loving, adventure-seeking, or community-driven. Perhaps it is humor, spirituality, or being a helper or a teacher. Whatever it is, this is where you must lay the foundation for your house of *committed* action. This is where your non-negotiable fitness habit becomes part of your blueprint, ingrained in your DNA, nestled in your soul.

The way you approach exercise is a choice. You can either begin your fitness routine thinking, "I *have* to do this," or, as I prefer, "I *get* to do this." When you *get* to work out, run, hike, swim, or whatever gets your heart pounding and body moving, you come from a place of gratitude and purpose. When you *have* to work out, you come from a place of fear, grasping, and obligation. Not that obligation is always a terrible thing, but it is important to remain clear about what it is that we are obligated to. Being obligated to feed and clothe your child is very different from feeling obligated to run for two hours every day, or to go to barre or spinning every day for a month, or even to hit a goal in a race if you are not really feeling it. Feeding and clothing your child is a real obligation, something you must do to live in alignment with your values. If you have children, you probably hold family as a very high value and work for your family's safety and welfare. Therefore, you will be committed to act: feeding your child is a *committed action* because it is driven by a value.

But why keep going on long runs or taking barre, if every time you tie your shoes or put on your sticky socks you think about how much you would rather be doing anything else? This is the problem with *having* to work out because of a goal or an obligation that you imposed on yourself, or that society imposed upon you. At the other side of that goal, there will be more goals, and more goals after that. There are no values driving you to act. You will probably not feel satisfied or remain committed after your goals have been met or when you tire of trying.

Sometimes goals are fine, but other times they detract from what would help you form a habit of fitness. The joy you feel when you live in alignment with your values is what will help you form a habit of fitness. We want to feel joy. If you find yourself *having* to work out, that is when it is time to become purpose-driven. Goals can also be purpose-driven if kept in perspective. Run that marathon, go for it! If you start to feel less and less excited about it, or if injuries pile up during your training, be willing to abandon ship. Because after all, what is the purpose of pursuing the goal?

Is the purpose increasing health so that you can continue to live aligned with your values?

When we are healthy, we live longer, and we can keep sharing our gifts. Your talents are your gifts, and the world needs you to share them—it really does! So perhaps being healthy allows you to live longer so that you can keep being an advocate for change in healthcare policy or education, because those things are aligned with your values. Now you can go into your fitness routine with the idea of I *get* to do this instead of I *have* to do this.

Fitness, like everything you encounter on your journey, can do one of two things: it can either support your life or your death. Yes, your death. Because the latter is the more off-putting statement, let us begin there. When you move from a place of obligation, from *having* to work out, the fitness routine will create stress in your life instead of much-needed stress relief. *Having* to work out can also sacrifice the actual needs of the body on the altar of the mind, leading to injury or burnout or worse: losing trust in your own innate knowing of what you need every day in an exercise or movement routine.

Here is an example: you are training for a marathon, and on Tuesday you have a nine-mile run planned, but you wake up with a creaky knee, having not slept because you had terrible dreams. Forcing action from a place of *having* to work out sends a message to the body that it is not safe with you, and eventually you will mute your body's signals more and more until its needs are a distant annoyance you cannot even make out anymore.

This does not mean there are not times where we need to push through resistance and build resilience, of course, for that is one of the greatest pearls daily exercise offers us. Resilience in the body will inevitably build resilience in the mind. What it does mean is that if we do not listen to our physiological needs and instead only focus on what our monkey mind is encouraging us to do, we can eventually lose control of the whole circus and forget how to hear what our bodies are telling us.

Before you go for your next workout, ask yourself two questions: "How do I feel today?" and "What do I need?" And finally, just as a litmus test, ask this bonus question: "Who is answering?" Maybe it is you answering, maybe it is your mother, maybe it is your friend or trainer, maybe it is a magazine you read at the grocery store. Be aware and only answer the calls of your self—after all, who knows you better than you? When we start to listen, we can start to come back to a place of gratitude, self-care, trust, and purpose-driven movement. When we do this, when we move with intention and inspiration tied together in a nice little bow and dusted with gratitude, exercise and fitness support our life. It makes us strong physically, emotionally, and psychologically. It keeps our heart pumping. It promises that we will be able to keep at our life's work longer than if we did not move, and that we will someday take our children's children's children swimming in the ocean when we are ninety-eight. It is a joyful experience and we *get* to do it. How lucky are we to be able to support our lives like this?

Carolee Walker says it perfectly: exercise is not an option. That is the truth. It is not an option. We all need to move our body. And to develop this non-negotiable, habitual state of action, we must keep coming back to our purpose, our source, that impalpable thing much bigger than any of us, that needs the magic and brilliance stored inside of all of us. We must return to the idea of action theory that we started with. We desire to be fit and healthy (who doesn't?), we believe that having a fitness routine will lead us to this fulfilled desire, so we are propelled into action, committed to getting our result—and to make this a lasting pattern, to propel ourselves into *committed action*, we stoke the fire with purpose.

You get to exercise, you do not have to. You get to. Let it be joyful. Do the things you love to do and leave behind the things that you do not. Run only downhill, dance in your living room with your dogs until you are sweaty, and listen to your favorite music while you hike. Commune with the experience of listening to yourself, harvesting awareness around how you feel and what you need, and begin to trust yourself on the deepest level of connectedness.

You get to exercise, you get to experience this life, you get to be resilient, and you have a purpose-driven life that needs you to keep on living it in a healthy, happy body.

And as Carolee would say, "You got this."

Sarajean Rudman
Glastonbury, Connecticut

INTRODUCTION

I've experienced two significant failures in my life.

Okay, I know that sounds dramatic. Let's just say I've made lots of mistakes over the years, but it's the two failures in my fifties that I want to focus on here. When I was younger, messing up didn't seem to sideline me. I was always back at it.

The first was in 2011, when I was fifty-three and I was on a detail assignment at the U.S. Department of State as a senior watch officer (SWO) in the Department's Operations Center.

SWOs have full command over the Department's official communications between principal officers and foreign government leaders. The workspace feels like a cockpit, but without the windows. SWOs flip a switch to activate a blue light when they need to step off the floor and use the bathroom. This is where SWOs live, sometimes for fourteen hours straight without a break. The shifts were one thing, but it often took two hours to read in and as long again to brief out. SWOs work overnight shifts, early morning shifts, and late afternoon shifts that end around midnight. I was tragically sleep-deprived and lacked the stamina to do the job.

I failed miserably and after two months curtailed from the assignment.

By the time I'd accepted the SWO assignment, which was prestigious, competitive, and critically important to the day-to-day workings of the U.S. government, I'd already enjoyed a full career, first as a public diplomacy writer and editor in the Bureau of Public Affairs, and later as a consular officer in the Bureau of Consular Affairs, assisting U.S. citizens overseas in emergencies. I was a coordinator on the Department's fast-paced task forces, often working overnight shifts, and was a chief point of contact, available 24/7, for the families of the hikers who were arrested and detained in Iran from 2009 to 2011.

So not cutting it as a SWO was a blow to my confidence that I've never completely shaken off.

Who knows whether I would have made a great SWO if I'd been in better physical shape, but even though my bureau welcomed me back with open arms, and my colleagues at the Operations Center assured me that good people curtail from assignments all the time, I spent the next two years questioning my ability to accomplish anything whatsoever.

In truth, it wasn't so much that I could not keep up physically that haunted me. It was my inability to bounce back. For me, the SWO problem had become all about the setback, and, in truth, it lingers.

My second failure was in September 2015, nearly a year and half after beginning my fitness journey, when I did not finish my first triathlon, the Bethany Beach Triathlon. I had made it through the ocean swim (nearly drowned) and finished the bike section (nearly got lost), but was disqualified before the run because of the race's strict time limits.

I was devastated. I felt I had let everyone down who'd supported me and trained me. Earlier the previous day, as I was loading my bike onto my Honda CRV outside my house before driving to the beach, a FedEx driver stopped on my street and jumped out of his truck.

"Can I help?" he asked.

"No, thank you," I replied as I turned to him.

"I got this."

That afternoon, as I drove to the beach, I was filled with excitement and dread all at the same time—just as I had been the day I walked into the Operations Center.

Now, as I lifted the bike onto the rack on the back of the CRV as we got ready to head home from the beach, I wondered why I thought I could complete a triathlon.

I know.

Really?

Putting failing as an SWO and failing to finish a race in the same category of failure?

So, here's the thing.

After a first-rate hamburger at the Dogfish Head Brewpub in Rehoboth and l e n g t h y conversations with my family about what I had done well during the race and what I needed to improve, within hours of emerging from that horrific ocean swim, I began the process of *failing forward*.

Of *bouncing back.*

Before turning in for bed that night, I wrote about what I had learned from the experience and submitted the piece to the *Huffington Post* Healthy Living editors for consideration. Earlier that month I had begun to publish my freelance wellness articles in the *Washington Post,* but I had followed Arianna Huffington's journey and was a fan of the *Huffington Post's* myriad and diverse contributors. By morning, as I was getting ready for work and turning my attention back to training for my first marathon in December 2015, I had received an invitation from the *Huffington Post* editors to join its team of wellness bloggers.

I sat at my kitchen island having coffee and closed my laptop.

"Wow," I must have said aloud, because my dog jumped up.

I was the editor in chief of *The Miscellany News* at Vassar, and I had spent the first two decades of my professional life doing some form of writing and editing, always planning a career as a journalist. Yet when I joined Consular Affairs, wondering whether I'd ever have the competitive edge or grit to make it in journalism, I did not think twice about putting aside my writing to learn something new.

It wasn't until March 2014 when I used my weight loss blog to hold myself accountable that I began to flex my writing muscles and discovered I had a passion for wellness subjects. If writing is about having something to say, here I was, after years away from a keyboard, with a lot on my mind.

Here's what's on my mind.

As I encounter challenges as I age and continually reinvent myself, I can't afford to let setbacks take me down. For me, running is hard, but every time I do it, for any length of time and for any distance, I simply feel better about myself.

Learning how to push myself, how to find my edge, how to stumble and recover—this is my foundation for becoming ageless, for being resilient. For bouncing back.

I'm not suggesting we have to run a marathon or be a triathlete, but we do need to become grounded in a meaningful exercise habit in order for exercise to matter. Every time I run I push myself physically, but mostly it's the mental effort that adds up. Each time, after each run, I am a little more empowered, a little more resilient. By discovering my edge, I'm in a better place to face the inevitable disappointments and obstacles with a comeback attitude.

Like I did when I was younger. When I was just a kid.

And not just after a run or a race.

In life.

***

When I lived in the San Francisco Bay Area in my early forties before joining the State Department, without a whole lot of drama going on in my life, I put on more than twenty pounds. I had never before been overweight and did not see the weight gain coming. My doctor ordered tests, but she knew what I knew—that at some time in a woman's forties, her metabolism changes.

"You're gaining weight because you're burning fewer calories than you're consuming."

Other words came to my mind.

Is this as good as it gets?

I was working as a freelance book editor, and since most of my clients were on the East Coast, I started my day at five in the morning but finished by two in the afternoon.

After the appointment with my doctor, I used my afternoons to rollerblade on a path overlooking San Francisco Bay in Foster City, met friends for hikes on Windy Hill or the Stanford Dish, and joined Weight Watchers. Within a few months I dropped more than twenty pounds.

We moved back to Washington, D.C., in 2005, when I started working at the Department of State as a writer and editor. I lost track of how long it took me to put that weight back on, but by the time my husband Bob and I were in London with a group of theatergoers from the Woolly Mammoth Theatre Company in February 2014, my mind-body connection was less than harmonious.

We were walking everywhere, seeing interesting shows with interesting people, and talking about theater.

But I felt like crap. I was huffing and puffing as I trudged through London's streets in the rain, and I was exhausted nearly all day. I was irritable and easily annoyed by anything outside my control, especially the relentless rain.

Bob had already been living and working during the week in a suburb outside Philadelphia before we came back from the trip, so I made a commitment to myself to figure out my weight gain and my constant feeling of exhaustion. At that time, I didn't acknowledge that I needed to establish a fitness habit. Back then I didn't even know there was such a thing.

When I tell you how ridiculously unprepared I was as I began this journey, try to imagine that I was even less well informed. In a lucky turn of fate, I connected with a gifted personal trainer half my age who agreed to ride along with me as we navigated a path to health and well-being.

Like many personal trainers, Reuel Tizabi, who left personal training to pursue physical therapy studies full time after working with me for nearly eleven months, had been an athlete with childhood dreams of playing professional sports. In Reuel's case, it was soccer.

Is this really happening? Reuel thought as the medics carried him off the soccer field on a stretcher after he suffered a tear to his anterior cruciate ligament (ACL), a common knee injury.

As Reuel told me his story, I didn't say anything. I was listening to him talk while he was trying to distract me during a wall sit, but I was thinking, *I've been there.* Once you hit your fifties, you've probably been there too.

Is this really happening?

With Reuel at the helm at first, and then by my side as an unexpected friend, I started training in the gym in the winter of 2014 and took up running to burn calories. By now I've run ten half-marathons, and I finished my first marathon in Negril, Jamaica, in December 2015. And, yes, I completed my first triathlon on June 12, 2016, in Cape Henlopen, Delaware.

What began as a journey to weight loss and getting fit turned into a path to self-confidence and wellness that has had an enormously positive impact on every aspect of both my personal life and my professional life. I fall asleep at night grateful for each day and wake up each morning full of optimism and good will.

Although I was a gymnast and a competitive swimmer as a teenager growing up on Long Island, I never considered myself an athlete. Until Title IX, schools and coaches rarely provided athletic guidance and support to girls' teams, and later, when I attempted to get fit, small injuries piled on top of each other like domino bones.

Yet even women who have been exercising for years face challenges when it comes to getting results. Often experts such as trainers and physicians enable us to take a comfortable approach to our fitness regimen because they do not take women seriously. Unless we had been athletes as kids or young adults, and few of us were, we do not know how to find our edge. Learning how to carve out time to meet our own fitness needs or how to "be the dog" and dig in, pushing ourselves physically and mentally, is one of the greatest challenges to aging well.

Since Day 1, I've continued to work with a series of first-rate personal trainers. And in another turn of fate, in the summer of 2015, when Dr. Katie Taraban Mahoney, my early physical therapist, left Washington to relocate to California, I met Dr. Kevin McGuinness, a sports medicine specialist at Washington Orthopedics and Sports Medicine. Kevin has put me back together after multiple small injuries and setbacks, and he is often a collaborator in my wellness writing. Kevin has helped me to enjoy becoming increasingly knowledgeable about the science of exercise, especially how exercise relates to aging well.

Early in 2016, I was taking a group exercise class at the gym when the teacher began, as many teachers do, by asking what was bothering us.

"Does anyone have any issues?"

I was used to thinking about these questions, especially in yoga, because I'm forever devising ways to modify poses.

"Knee problems?"

"Raise your hand if you've got back issues!"

"Hips?"

I looked around the studio, and I was surrounded by a super-fit, ultra-fashionable group of women. Even so, there were a lot of hands in the air.

The instructor, Jennifer Blackburn, was wearing a Madonna-style wireless headset, and her voice dominated the room, even above Flo Rida's "Low," which I remember was playing because oddly, the song had popped up on my mix during my morning run. I instinctively touched my ears to see if I was somehow still wearing my wireless earbuds.

"This is the year you want to fix that."

I have some ideas why it can take more than a sea change in a regular woman's life for her to develop a serious exercise routine. Off the top of my head, raising children often plays havoc with any routine, let alone a healthy one. When my children were young, it was a good day if I shaved both legs in the same shower.

This is the year you want to fix that.

But another challenge is addressing all of our little issues that have a way of distracting us and diminishing our self-confidence or level of endurance. I remember early in my training in 2014, Katie stared me straight in the eye and told me my knee was FINE. I'm using caps because she was kind of yelling at me.

Two years earlier, an orthopedic surgeon had removed 70 percent of the meniscus around my left knee, and every time I got out of a deep chair (squat) or bent down to pick up the morning paper (lunge) since then, I felt that bone-on-bone sensation you read about.

"Your knee is fine," Katie said, exasperated. "YOU'RE FINE."

Katie showed me how to strengthen the muscles and tissues around my knee so I could exercise vigorously, including running. I still do these exercises, and finally in 2016, under Kevin's guidance, I added actual squats and lunges to my regimen. Both of these exercises are fundamental for strengthening the glutes, which is at this point also critical to achieving nearly all of my fitness goals.

So here is what I want to say about getting in shape.

We can't accomplish anything until we (1) address and fix our issues, and (2) establish a meaningful fitness habit.

Over the past three years, I have rarely had a clear sense of when I needed to deal with an issue or put it aside, so I know this isn't easy or simple. If my shoulder was bothering me, I skipped the pool and focused on running or cycling. If my knee felt wonky, I stopped running and was back in the pool.

In our everyday lives, this kind of working around problems is a good thing. We're creative and flexible and we're efficient at getting things done any way we can.

But in terms of our health and well-being, we need to figure out why our knees hurt and fix them. Sure, we may still need to work around them and bike instead of run, but at least we'll know what it is we need to do and make a plan.

Because exercise is not optional.

You don't need me to tell you that becoming fit in middle age is critical to preventing or at least putting off some of the most common serious medical diseases as we age, including Alzheimer's and dementia, cardiovascular disease, diabetes, and many types of cancer. These stories pop into our social media newsfeeds nearly every day.

As women, we talk a lot about what we want. We want to lose weight. We want more energy. We want better jobs. We want tighter skin. What we should be talking about, in the words of legendary coach Dan John, is what we need to do to achieve any of this.

For me that means that on a regular basis I'm finding myself in a room with a sports medicine specialist, as well as a physical therapist who understands my need and desire to be active. I'm continuing to learn about strength training from my trainers and also from Kevin, because he has me addressing and fixing my issues one by one.

The idea is that the better we get at exercising by addressing and fixing our issues, the more we'll hate it less and ultimately begin to take real pleasure in the activity.

I began my fitness journey in earnest in 2014, and as I look back it occurs to me that my greatest achievement then was what I needed most: to develop a serious fitness habit.

Developing a habit was not what I wanted.

What I wanted was results.

If Reuel had said, "Actually, your goal is to develop a fitness habit," I'm sure I would have been outta there.

Yet this idea is backed up by numerous scientific studies that point out that in order for exercise to matter, it needs to be frequent, intense, and vigorous.

According to a December 31, 2015, *Washington Post* Op Ed, "The Five Myths of Our Habits," it takes an average of sixty-six days to form a new habit. While some simple behaviors may only need to be repeated for a few weeks in order for you to continue doing them without thinking about it, some, like exercise, can take a year.

A year.

A freakin' year.

The author, Wendy Wood, a University of Southern California psychologist, suggested that setting a routine (what you do to get ready or prepare) may be even more critical to forming a habit than repetition (exercising). Even now, I plan out my week, incorporating my exercise and nutrition into my work schedule, I set out my workout clothes before I go to sleep, and I am out the door to run or train by 5:15 a.m. I don't think about it. It's like brushing my teeth, which is what I do *after* drinking coffee, not before—another mindless ritual.

By this point, I may be obsessed with my fitness routine, but like my coffee addiction, I'm good with that, because the benefits are worth it. I take true pleasure in the moments in my day when I'm moving around.

The point is to get set in a fitness habit and schedule your workouts in the same way you factor in anything else you need to do every day. What's important, according to Wood, is that whatever we do, it needs to become routine. If you can only exercise three mornings per week, establish a routine for this until it becomes a habit.

And here's where establishing a fitness habit gets so challenging, and possibly why many of us are setting the same fitness goals year after year.

What if you don't enjoy exercising? Or what if you are like me when I started and so out of shape that exercising is physically and mentally uncomfortable?

My niece Nina Lish, an architecture student in Philadelphia, told me about a podcast she heard on "Freakonomics" with Katherine Milkman called "When Willpower Isn't Enough." Milkman, who coined the phrase "temptation bundling," suggests that if we can combine two activities—one you should do but tend to avoid, and one you love to do but that may not be entirely productive—we can have better success achieving our goals.

The example she gave is this one: Milkman hates to exercise and loves to watch television when she's got other important things to do. She told herself she could only watch her favorite shows when she was at the gym, so after a few evenings, she found herself rushing to get to the gym.

"Or like having a beer while you fold the laundry," Nina said.

"Was that an example in the podcast?" I asked.

Gretchen Rubin, author of *The Happiness Project*, writes about this in her book *Better Than Before*. Like Milkman, Rubin, who doesn't focus on exercise, makes the case for combining activities in order to form a habit. So genius, but not so different from gradually loading your child's plate of beige foods with colorful, healthy items. We've all done that, right?

As I began to develop my exercise habit, without thinking about it and without seeing fast results, music became my incentive to work out. It occurred to me that as I had my children and worked outside the home, I never noticed how much music had fallen by the wayside. If you ask me what I most look forward to on a long run, I'd have to put listening to music high up in the plus column. Now I devote a chunk of time on a regular basis to catching up on new artists as I curate and build my music playlists for exercising as well as warming up and stretching.

"You have the music taste of a fifteen-year-old," my State Department colleague and friend Steve Royster told me after he came across my blog and playlists and agreed to read an early draft of this manuscript.

Ha, I smiled. *You have no idea.*

It's not just my taste in music, which by the way is closer to that of a thirty-year-old. It's my brain, too. It's as if by developing a meaningful exercise habit and discovering my edge, I've found a way to live all of my ages at once. Kind of like being fifteen—or thirty, but with the benefit of being fifty-something.

I'm good with that.

＊＊＊

I was in New York City in July 2016 attending the opening of the New York Music Festival as my daughter, Mia Walker, and my son, Adin Walker, made their New York professional debut working together as director and choreographer, respectively. I asked the concierge in my midtown hotel if she could recommend a good place for my morning run. After she mapped out my route to the High Line, she put down her pen and sighed.

"I wish I could be a runner," she said.

"You can," I quickly responded.

"Look at you," she said. "You're so fit."

We talked for a few minutes about the importance of making time for ourselves, of starting out slowly and committing to walking a few blocks every day.

"Seriously, if I can do this, you can," I said. I showed her my before-and-after photo, and she nodded.

"You got this," I said.

And you can, too

NOTE TO THE READER

What follows are posts from my original blog, SKINNYCAROLEE, which was hosted on BlogSpot from February 2014 until August 2015. I started my journey with a goal of transforming my physical appearance, but when I made the transition from focusing on losing weight to learning how to carve out time to meet my own fitness needs and to push myself physically and mentally, I moved the blog over to my personal website hosted by Squarespace and renamed it BE THE DOG.

Awesome people you'll meet throughout this book:

Adin – My insanely artistic son, a dancer and athlete, who's always there to encourage me to dig in.

Adorable – Reuel Tizabi, my original trainer at Equinox Bethesda who's on his way to receiving his doctor of physical therapy degree.

Buff – Shoubry Sos, my trainer at Equinox Bethesda after Reuel left to return to school full time.

Lord Baltimore – Bob Walker, my husband, who was born and raised royally in Baltimore.

Mia – My wildly talented daughter, who heads up my squad and who sensibly reminds me when I get anxious before a race, "Mom, you volunteered for this."

MCRRC – Montgomery County Road Runners Club.

Patrick Gatti – An American businessman on assignment in Kingston who ran with me in Emancipation Park in the evenings after work and talked endlessly with me about my upcoming first half marathon, D.C. Rock 'n' Roll.

Perfectly Nice – Daniel Le, my trainer at Equinox Bethesda when Reuel attended the World Cup in Brazil.

Really Smart – Dr. Katie Taraban Mahoney, my physical therapist at Elite Physical Therapy and Wellness Center in Washington, D.C., who relocated to the San Francisco Bay Area in 2015.

Ripped – Neile Miller, my Vassar classmate who also trained with Reuel.

Triathlete – My good friend and work colleague, who's apparently naturally athletic.

Wonderful – Francis Bass, my massage therapist, who has sadly relocated out of Washington, D.C.

CHAPTER 1 – OMG—ENDORPHINS ARE FOR REAL

Day 1, March 30, 2014

> *"We're running around like we're brainless."*
> —Rizzle Kicks, "Down with the Trumpets"

I was never a gym person. The whole gym culture had run right past me. My family has always belonged to a local health club, and Bob, my husband, Lord Baltimore, and Mia and Adin, my adult children, work out at the gym as often as they can. My father, Len Belkin, walks daily and swims twice a week. They've all got a gym routine that I somehow never felt I needed. I had lots of excuses. I wanted to be home with Mia and Adin in the evenings when they were in middle and high school. Later, when they were barely home themselves, I needed to rush through the front door to feed the dog. And I had cooking to do.

I had begun to practice yoga around 2011, and in late 2013, I joined Equinox in Bethesda for the early morning yoga classes. I developed a particular fondness for the club's yoga studio, which is outfitted with individually operated ceiling fans, so if you arranged things optimally you could set yourself directly underneath one and ask the teacher to turn it on.

When I returned from a theater trip to London in February 2014 and felt limited by my lack of energy, I agreed to meet with one of the Equinox trainers who had been emailing me incessantly offering a free fitness assessment and a free personal training session.

I had ignored these emails and put off the training team for an incredibly long time.

A few days after returning from London, I met Reuel Tizabi, an adorable trainer, at Equinox Bethesda after work. I—*ahem*—had forgotten to bring my sneakers, so we would be *limited* in what we could do during the assessment.

I stepped on the scale, and I weighed 121 pounds. I know that doesn't sound like a lot to you, but I'm 4'10" and my ideal weight is closer to 95 pounds, so that's a lot of extra weight on my small frame.

Wow, when did that happen? He went through everything else: pulse rate, body fat index, *blah blah blah,* I wasn't paying attention—121 pounds?

I agreed to the free personal training session with Adorable. He told me to arrive 10 minutes early so I could warm up on the treadmill, and he would meet me there. In the meantime, before the first training session, I came across the latest issue of *More* magazine, which featured the fifty-nine-year-old author of the book *Labor Day,* who began a weight loss and fitness regimen at the San Francisco Equinox. I read the article and handed Adorable the magazine. By the time we met for the second time, Adorable was referring to the flabby personalities under my arms as "Aunt Betty."

The initial training sessions were astoundingly difficult and embarrassing. No matter what we did, I was completely out of breath and lightheaded. Did I say I was embarrassed? Adorable could tell when I needed to take a lap around the training area—he'd walk with me, and I would feel even more on display as an overweight miniature dinosaur. It's amazing that I never ran into anyone I knew at Equinox. I live in Bethesda. Kind of a miracle. Kind of amazing I never ran into anyone, literally.

I told Adorable I had a dress I wanted to wear to the Woolly Mammoth Theater Company Gala in two weeks. It was the one I had planned to wear to the Tony Awards the previous year as Mia's guest when *Pippin* was nominated for a bunch of Tonys—but I had worn Option B, which was black and forgiving. Adorable was straightforward. He told me I would not see results by then, but he reminded me I was in this for the long haul. We would work Aunt Betty hard.

"You'll see results in sixteen weeks," he said.

After a week of training with Adorable I had difficulty buttoning my suit jacket around my chest, and I had gained three pounds. I told Adorable about *those* results.

This was good information, he noted, because that gave him important insight into how he wanted to move forward. At my request, we stopped using weights and began increasing the number of repetitions using resistance bands. He told me to come in as much as possible to walk on the treadmill, and we were working to strengthen the area around my left knee since I had never done what my then-physical therapist told me to do after my knee surgery in September 2012. "There's only so much progress you can make if you can't get your knee to stabilize," Adorable said.

"It's not about losing weight," Adorable told me as he looked at me directly. "It's about how you feel and about being healthy and fit."

"It's about losing weight," I said. "Like about twenty pounds."

I had already searched the internet and found that weight gain was a common side effect of working out for the first time. So I told myself I'd be okay with this for now and see how it went.

Those first mornings on my own on the treadmill seemed pointless. I wore baggy sweatpants and an oversize T-shirt. I brought a mug of coffee. And everything hurt. Adorable told me to go at any pace as long as I got in at least two miles. That was about 90 minutes of walking. It took me nearly 45 minutes to walk a single mile.

At first, I watched the news on the big screens in the second-floor training rooms, but as I upped my speed and my distance, I turned to the playlists on my iPhone for inspiration.

I went to R & J Sports in Bethesda, and they put me in Brooks running shoes that were, I'm not exaggerating, like walking on a cloud. They also sold me a pair of ultrathin Balega socks that absolutely do not slip, so I finally said goodbye to two blistering blisters. I picked up some Under Armour slightly fitted short sleeve T-shirts that didn't stick to me, as odd as that sounds. For my legs, even now I am convinced my Lululemon yoga pants are the best things on the planet. I read about the controversy over those pants a few years ago, but there is simply nothing like them. Even now I rinse them out more frequently than I'd like, but remember I was working with Adorable, who stood very close to me for 60 minutes and stared at every move I made.

I suspect it's an occupational hazard for trainers if they've got to work that closely with people who do not rinse out their yoga pants.

At one of our earliest sessions, Adorable asked me if I felt the burn after we did 20 reps focusing on my glutes.

"What would make you think I wouldn't feel the burn?" I asked.

"Just checking."

Adorable told me some clients prefer that he count every repetition aloud. We didn't work that way. I'd usually ask him where we were when I thought I was out of oxygen.

My favorite words: "Five more." My least favorite: "Eleven more."

When we were focusing on my core, wherever that was, I looked over at Adorable, and I'm sure he was thinking he was glad the Equinox Fitness Training Institute includes CPR certification. As good as he is, it would probably not be helpful to his career to kill one of his clients.

There was a session around that time where it was all I could do to keep from throwing up right there in the gym. I struggled on the drive home, and when I arrived at my house, I wasn't sure if I should call 911.

But that night I went to sleep and felt fine when my alarm went off at 5:00 a.m. I walked into my gym clothes with that sense of euphoria that you read about. *I am on the other side of this.*

That was when we began to have regular discussions about the difference between pain and burn. There was no safe answer to his question, "Are you feeling pain or burn?" If I said pain (especially if it related to my lower back), we would simply stop immediately and move to that horrible machine that works your lower back until you feel the burn.

Day 2, March 31, 2014

> *"Yeah baby, it hurts a bunch*
> *The girls got going and we had a munch*
> *I promise on a dime, it's the last time*
> *I'll never have a liquid lunch."*
>
> —Caro Emerald, "Liquid Lunch"

I tried to cram in as much cardio as I could this morning. I would have done more if I didn't need to shower and dress for work. I walked nearly four miles on the treadmill; for the first three miles I was walking briskly at 3.6 MPH, and for the last almost-mile, I walked at 3.7 MPH. After the treadmill, I did five minutes on the arm bike, which was all I had time for, but more importantly, it was as much as I could take.

Most of this morning's music came from my Ladies Night mix, the one I'm compiling in anticipation of my annual Ladies Night Out in December. I came across "Liquid Lunch" by Caro Emerald from *The Shocking Miss Emerald* album. I must have Shazamed it when I was shopping for my nieces and nephews during the holidays at H & M in Georgetown. And this one: "You Just Don't Love Me" from David Morales. Shameless techno club pushed me through my last six or seven minutes.

I'd gotten in the habit of bringing my coffee with me to the gym in the mornings. This started when I was taking yoga classes at six o'clock in the morning. I know it's not very Zen to have coffee in the studio or very smart to hydrate with coffee during cardio workouts, but at least in those early weeks the coffee kept me from sliding off the back of the treadmill. My childhood BFF Ken Levitan, the country music mogul and foodie in Nashville, will appreciate this, because he was the one who told me he knows how to sneak coffee into the Ashram in Los Angeles. My apologies if it wasn't you, Ken. I wouldn't want to get you in trouble.

After work, I took a yin yoga class with Christopher Brown. Yin is my favorite yoga practice, and I look forward to taking this class whenever possible. We hold poses deeply and for a long time, so you can feel the stretch in the joints as well as in the muscles. Christopher says to find the place between too much and not enough first physically and then mentally, and stay there. It's so interesting how different my mind works when I'm in the zone during a training session versus being completely present during a yin practice. As a type-A New Yorker, it took a significant effort to get the "being present" concept in yoga. When I'm in the zone during a training session, my mind goes to the strangest kaleidoscopic mix of places—from the Clinique counter at Lord and Taylor to any aisle at Strosniders hardware store.

Nutrition

Pre-cardio: one half Ozery Onebun (wholegrain) with Smart Balance margarine and orange marmalade

Breakfast: whole wheat English muffin with a dollop of fat-free cottage cheese

Morning snack: fat-free Greek yogurt and berries

Lunch: salad with homemade baked tofu and a sliced apple.

I'm going to date myself here to share my secret for baked tofu, which comes from the original Moosewood cookbook. If you're in a hurry, which I frequently am, you can just slice the tofu (I use lite extra firm when I can find it, otherwise, regular extra firm) and marinate it for at least 30 minutes in the Moosewood concoction or your own sesame/soy mixture. Most of the time, if I'm taking this approach, I prefer Soy Vay Hawaiian style. Just cover the bottom of a lasagna pan with a small amount of the marinade and let the tofu slices sit for 30 minutes (flipping the pieces over after 15 minutes). Then bake in a 350-degree oven for 30 minutes. Once cooled, you can transfer to a storage bowl and keep in the fridge for a few days. The slices make great sandwiches with light mayo and lettuce and tomato on pita or whole wheat or tossed in salads.

Afternoon snack: Nutrigrain bar (yeah, I know I can do better than that) and a cup of green tea.

Dinner: Because by now it was nearly 9 p.m., I passed on the impulse to pour a bowl of cereal. I had a piece of grilled fish and some roasted cauliflower and Brussels sprouts left over from the weekend.

My plan was to get on the scale in a few days, so I was crossing my fingers that the numbers would go down or at least not up.

Day 3, April 1, 2014

*"Bring your body and let me switch up
your atmosphere."*
—Flo Rida, "Club Can't Handle Me"

The fifty-nine-year-old writer in the *More* magazine feature training at the San Francisco Equinox talked about how out of place she felt among the otherwise well-dressed, well-appointed, and well-preserved men and women working out around her. What got me when I looked around the training room in Bethesda was not so much how out of style I felt—although there was that—it was how out of step I was. Right from the treadmill, where serious people-watching is matched only by passing an afternoon at a Parisian café, I was impressed by the large number of clients working with trainers and on their own to maintain their physical health. Sure, there were a few like me who were starting at square one, but remarkably few. I began to recognize Adorable's clients, since he would greet them warmly while he was working with me, and later, when we saw each other on our own, we would share a pleasantry. We were all writing the same page from a similar chapter in our unique personal stories.

Triathlete was getting ready to train for a race over the summer, and she casually began to plan her workouts and diet. She had done this before, so she was in a position where she could afford to let her discipline slide. I wasn't so slick. Over the years I had let everything go, and I knew I was looking at months of meticulously scheduled workouts.

I felt defeated when Adorable stopped me after five reps when I wanted to do ten more. He didn't do it often, but when he did, I got the message.

"Why are you being so hard on yourself?" Triathlete asked me.

"Look at all this time and work ahead of me," I said. "I'm so stupid."

Nutrition

It wasn't a great food day. During our early morning session Adorable had pointed out that without something to burn, without fuel, I'd poop out, which I did. I'm sure he used a more scientific description to make his point, but I was recovering from our third set of core work and had only absorbed the gist of what he was trying to communicate. After the session, I had to get ready for work quickly, and the morning flew by. I did not have time to eat my morning yogurt and fruit and only had time to manage half of my salad. At a social event I had a beer and a potato pierogi and then headed to the gym for cardio.

By the time I met Triathlete for dinner at Lebanese Taverna in Bethesda, I was coasting on fumes. We shared some mezza—mostly vegetarian—and I said no to a glass of wine. I was glad I was committed to staying focused, because otherwise I might have had two beers in the afternoon and joined Triathlete for a glass of wine with dinner. Even with only having picked up every other word, I figured that was not the fuel Adorable had in mind.

🎵 PLAYLIST HIGHLIGHTS

Pre-training Warm Up

Go Do – Jonsi

Viva la Vida – Coldplay

Somewhere Only We Know – Keane

After-work Cardio
(3.88 miles / 65 minutes / mostly 3.7 MPH)

Pumped it up tonight—I needed it.

Timber – Pitbull

Coastin' – Zion I and K. Flay

Down With The Trumpets – Rizzle Kicks

You're No Good – Major Lazer

Right Round – Flo Rida (My all-time favorite.)

Envy – 116 Man Up (I love this riff on Bernadette Peters and Tom Wopat in the 1999 Tony award winning revival of *Annie Get Your Gun*, which featured Mia as Nellie Oakley—you can hear her on the Broadway cast recording.)

Rough Water – Travie McCoy

Club Can't Handle Me – Flo Rida (This was also playing during our training session just when I thought I was about to go bust—it got me through.)

Cool Down

m.A.A.d city – Kendrick Lamar (Explicit, but incredibly narrative, and a good six-minute focus piece.)

Day 4, April 2, 2014

> *"Just because it burns."*
> —Pink, "Try"

There are moments when I think there are so many parts of my body that need an overhaul that if I could concentrate on fixing one part at a time, the process might seem more productive. I bet when Adorable met me for the first time and considered how he would approach our fitness regimen, he must have felt like a college student looking around his room in the middle of the semester.

Where to begin.

We were catching up that morning and going over my plan for nontraining days, and it struck me how strategic fitness training is. I'm the last to find out the plan for a training session, which is okay by me, but if a trainer begins each session as if it's the first time you've worked together or who wants to try out something new in the gym, you need to move on. I have little goals and big goals, and that's where the strategy part comes in. I think that's why Adorable said it takes 16 weeks of intensely working out to see results; you can't work everything at the same time. Bummer, I know! Wouldn't it be nice to see your arms slim down after pumping 30 leg lifts?

My little goals are to build stamina and to go shopping in my closet. My big goals are to go running on the Capital

Crescent Trail and to let the sun see as much of my skin as is legally acceptable without embarrassing Mia and Adin.

I had to be at work for an early meeting, so I did a quick workout. I didn't do any yoga that evening, since I was co-hosting a Meet the Candidate Dessert at my house with Jordan Cooper, Democratic Maryland General Assembly Candidate representing District 16, a fellow Vassar College alum. My guilty pleasure was a single slice of chocolate babka from Green's of Brooklyn.

🎵 PLAYLIST HIGHLIGHTS

Warm Up

Try – Pink

Monster – Eminem

Before-work Cardio

(3 miles / 45 minutes / 3.7 MPH; arm bike 5 minutes).

Blurred Lines – Glee cast version (Don't judge.)

I Am the Best – 2NE1 (Adin sent me this one.)

Get Lucky – Daft Punk

Stronger – Kanye

Sunshine – Mos Def

Crazy Kids – Kesha

American Idiot – Green Day

Cool down

The Boxer – Mumford and Sons version

Fare Thee Well – Mumford and Sons

Day 5, April 3, 2014

"Tell it like it is"
—Aaron Neville, "Tell It Like It Is"

I weighed in at 120 pounds, an official loss of a single pound since late February. I was mildly discouraged and bummed but not surprised. My goal was to use the weekend to think through and prepare the kind of food I would need to eat moving forward. Adorable encouraged me to consult a registered dietician. I knew I needed to find the right balance of protein in my diet since I have a natural tendency to bulk up. My focus for now would be complex carbs, including fruit and vegetables.

Training with Adorable that evening was more difficult than I anticipated. And it was practically always difficult. I would try to tell you what we worked on, but as at the time I did not know a single thing about exercise science or anatomy, I'll simply note that I thought we were working on my core, but learned later we were strengthening the muscles around my knees.

***

It's not that I am not self-aware about how mundane a lot of what I am writing might sound to many people, especially friends who have taken significant steps to stay in good physical shape for years. I also know my musings about my training sessions may often sound stupid, but I promise I am not posing as someone I am not. I *am* stupid. I still reach for a "Slow Start" button every time I step onto the treadmill, expecting to find it right next to the "Quick Start" one that I need to tap three times before it agrees to get going.

The irony is not lost on me that when I first came in to the Department of State as a public diplomacy writer for the former website www.america.gov (now www.share. america.gov), from the beginning I covered First Lady Michelle Obama's kitchen garden and her kids' healthy eating/Let's Move campaign. Although my colleagues knew I kept signing up for the beat just to get another glimpse of dreamy White House kitchen chef Sam Kass, I—like whole continents of women—admired Michelle Obama's unambiguous commitment to keeping herself in awesome shape. I never said it aloud, but it crossed my mind even then that she must have a strategy for staying fit while making room on her full plate for fruits and vegetables, running on the treadmill, and advocacy for veterans and military families.

🎵 PLAYLIST HIGHLIGHTS

Warm Up

Tainted Love – Soft Cell (This one stayed with me all day.)

Electric Avenue – Eddy Grant (From Killer on the Rampage.)

Before-work cardio
(4 miles! Over 60 minutes / 3.7 MPH)

My Evolving Beach Mix:

I Don't Wanna Dance – Eddy Grant

Drop Baby Drop – Eddy Grant

Exodus – Bob Marley

Many Rivers to Cross – Jimmy Cliff

You Can Get It If You Really Want – Jimmy Cliff (Of course.)

Tell It Like It Is – Aaron Neville

Electric Avenue extended Version – Eddy Grant (Probably on repeat twice—I'm old school with a time-honored passion for reggae/calyso/zydeco.)

No cool down this morning as I was in too much of a hurry to get to work. It's a good thing I like my job.

Day 6, April 5, 2014

> *"Leave those umbrellas at home."*
> —The Weather Girls, "It's Raining Men"

I had woken up fighting a cold, which I likely caught at the gym. I'm not complaining. Equinox is extremely well-kept, with members who regularly wipe off the machines both before and after using them. Trainers walking the floor are constantly bringing around clean hand towels, including chilled towels soaked in eucalyptus, and in the yoga studio you rarely see body fluids pooled on the floor. It's like when your child goes to day care for the first time. My children were always bringing home bugs that made a run at me even when, over time, the kids seemed immune.

Despite the periodic club emails reminding members of basic etiquette, you know there will always be that person. I'd seen her at the gym a few Saturdays in a row. She was probably in her fifties and in extremely good shape. She would come in from a run outside and settle her things, including a duffle and a designer handbag, next to the elliptical machine outside the restroom door. She would begin to strip off her outdoor running clothes and add them to the pile of bags on the floor. She would tap her running shoes to shake off the mud, and then she'd stack several newspapers on the machine. As she exercised and made her way through the papers, she'd toss the pages one by one to the floor on all sides of the machine. Other members nimbly stepped over the pile of clothing and bags, the discarded pages, and the dirt to reach the restroom and other machines.

The first time I observed this routine, especially during the disrobing, I was sure there was a *Candid Camera* crew somewhere. Then I wondered whether I had missed a Groupon offering discounted membership if you didn't use the lockers, which, by the way, have wooden hangers.

My take is you have to be at a certain phase in your life to appreciate working out in a civilized environment. I'm sure at another point in time, this would have been a turn off. Now I craved it.

Usually when I've finished a workout, especially in the early mornings before work, I would get into my car energized and alert. But occasionally, as on that morning, I might feel lightheaded and disoriented. I was able to add 10 minutes to my workout because I walked to two different parking lots before I remembered I had parked on the street directly in front of the gym. I walked by my car twice heading for the lots.

"Is this something you plan to bring up with your physician?" Lord Baltimore asked me, not so much as a question but as a commentary.

Cardio

I walked three miles at 3.7 MPH and did five minutes maintaining 60 RPM on the arm bike. Then I finished up on the mat with planks and a few core favorites, and of course straight-leg lifts.

🎵 PLAYLIST HIGHLIGHTS

I shuffled between a bunch of interesting mixes I'd created over the years, and the result was a little chaotic but definitely fun.

Warm up

It's Raining Men – The Weather Girls

In Da Club – 50 Cent

Cardio

My Evolving Ladies Night Mix: **Some old, some new.**

Keep Breathing – Ingrid Michaelson

Set Fire to the Rain – Adele

Paper Planes – M.I.A.

Count on Me – Bruno Mars

Where Does the Good Go – Tegan and Sara

Whatcha Say – Jason Derulo

God Only Knows – Beach Boys

Mad World – Michael Andrews/Gary Jules—from Donnie Darko

Team – Lorde

Brave – Sara Bareilles

Cool Down

Some Nights – Fun.

Oh What a World – Rufus Wainwright

Day 9, April 7, 2014

"A dream's a dream"
—Jack Johnson, "Dreams Be Dreams"

Around this time last year, my father-in-law, Roland Walker, died. Before he was diagnosed with Lou Gehrig's disease (ALS), which he battled for eighteen months, he was a savvy criminal defense attorney in Baltimore. He turned eighty-three in the fall of 2013 but embodied the phrase, "Eighty is the new sixty." He was an avid cyclist, and he worked out daily in the gym he had built in his Baltimore home. As ALS began to take away his ability to walk or to move his arms, he used his courtroom charm to persuade his Johns Hopkins physician to prescribe physical therapy. The physician told him to think through whether physical therapy was the right approach.

"If it makes you feel better, then do it," the doctor told him. "If it tires you out and saps your energy so you're unable to spend time with your family, then I wouldn't recommend it. Physical therapy will not help you walk or hold things in your hand."

Tough words. No one was surprised when Roland refused to accept this as his reality and set up his PT appointments. By the time he struggled to inhale his last gulps of air, he had lived many months beyond the average ALS patient of his age.

It's not a stretch to reason that he lasted as long as he did because he took care to stay in shape throughout his later years.

It was Roland who introduced me to the incredible Northern Central Railroad bike trail in Monkton. He befriended the owner of the local bike shop and convinced him to let him store his gear so he wouldn't have to lug it around in his two-seater. His enthusiasm for boxing, football, biking, fishing, and exercising in general was infectious, and I think I can speak for his children and their spouses when I suggest most of our biking trips— and probably all of our fishing trips—were Roland's idea. He wasn't much of a baseball fan, but he liked me, so if I bought the tickets to Camden Yards, he'd go.

A few days before Roland's death, when we all knew it was close to the end, one of his daughters, my sister-in-law Nicole Upton, made a commitment to herself to get fit and lose weight. By now, Nicole has lost 52 pounds, and her goal is to lose 20 more. In a similar way to what I had been doing, she devised a workout and diet regimen and held herself accountable by following through every single day. The results are absolutely amazing. She acknowledges how hard it's been but how much she continues to value the payoff. Nicole was one of the people who inspired me to get serious.

Adorable and I had a brief conversation about inspiration versus motivation. Some clients—not just his—want a trainer to motivate them, he said. This approach to training is common in the military. Think drill sergeant.

I am inspired by people, music, art, I said. What motivates me is *moi*.

Over the weekend I shopped for and prepared meals I wanted to have ready to go. For afternoon snacks, I made granola from Cannell et Vanille with changes and additions kitchen-tested by my sister-in-law Susan Walker. In addition to being absolutely fantastic and enlightened, the cinnamony smells linger for almost as long as a piece of salmon cooked on the stove. I've been making this granola for my family ever since Susan shared it with me. Unfortunately, I developed a sudden allergy to nuts, so while I continue to make this granola, I'm sadly not the one who gets to enjoy it, unless I swap out the almonds and pistachios for peanuts.

Whenever possible, I'm using my weekends to roast seasonal vegetables. My favorites are beets, Brussels sprouts, cauliflower, baby eggplant, broccoli, and bell peppers. For lunches, I add these to greens and my baked tofu or leftover grilled fish.

I've started to pick up clementines for snacking after work and before yoga or training.

For dinners, I've made Channa Masala a staple in my repertoire, and I'm serving it with wilted kale, collard, mustard greens, and whatever yogurt sauce I can whip together on top of half a piece of whole wheat naan. (The Channa Masala recipe is adapted from chef Rupen Rao from an Indian cooking class I took with Lord Baltimore and my sister Ilene Lish, along with her husband, Ethan Lish. The recipe is also on the side of the box of the Channa Masala spice tin.) This is so good and easy to make. Some of the Indian spices are hard to find, but Rupen Rao sells his spice collections online, which is helpful.

In the mornings before workouts, I've replaced the slice of toast with a banana and a small glass of freshly squeezed orange juice made the old-fashioned way with a hand juicer, so I'm getting the juice, pulp, and even some seeds. I'm crossing my fingers that the vitamin C will help me fend off a threatening cold. So far, no traces of a bug, although the seeds may be lingering. (TMI?)

Tomorrow is a training day. I'm glad I had three days to recover from Friday's early morning session, because I did not feel the full effect of what we did until Sunday. I guess it takes a few days for traumatized connective tissues to secrete fluid and become inflamed. Impressed?

Tonight, I worked to find that sweet spot in Christopher's yin yoga class.

"But if you work too hard to find it, you can't enjoy it; if you don't work hard enough, you lose focus and your mind wanders."

Christopher is like the Yoda of yin. Roland would have been so into him.

ENLIGHTENED GRANOLA

Adapted from Cannell et Vanille

Ingredients

3 cups extra-thick rolled oats

1½ cups nuts and seeds. I use a combination of slivered almonds, pistachios, sunflower seeds, pumpkin seeds, and unsweetened shredded coconut

½ cup apple juice

½ cup maple syrup

¼ cup olive oil

2 Tbsp. pure vanilla extract

½ tsp. ground cinnamon

1 tsp. fine sea salt

1½ cup dried fruit. I use raisins, dried cranberries, dried blueberries, and dried strawberries, if I can find them.

Instructions

1. Preheat oven to 325 degrees Fahrenheit (160 degrees Celsius).

2. Combine the oats, nuts, and seeds in a large bowl.

3. Combine the apple juice, maple syrup, olive oil, vanilla extract, cinnamon, and sea salt in a small bowl.

4. Pour the liquid over the dry ingredients and toss to coat.

5. Spread the mixture evenly on a baking sheet coated with parchment paper.

6. Bake for 40 minutes until golden. Stir the mixture after 20 minutes to make sure it is evenly baked.

7. Let the granola cool completely. It will become crunchier as it sits.

8. Stir in the dried fruit when completely cool.

9. Store in an airtight container.

CHANNA MASALA CURRY
Adapted from Rupen Rao

Ingredients

4 Tbsp. olive oil

1 cup minced red onion

2 cups canned garbanzo beans, rinsed

1 Tbsp. minced ginger

1 Tbsp. minced garlic

1 can diced tomatoes, including juice

Spice mix:
(You can also buy Rupen's Channa Masala spice mix. The recipe is on the tin, so it tells you how much to use.)

1 Tbsp. yellow curry powder

1 tsp. garam masala powder

1 tsp. mango powder

½ tsp. cayenne powder

Salt to taste

½ fresh lemon juice

Chopped cilantro

Instructions

1. In a skillet, heat the oil over medium heat.

2. Add onions and sauté for 5 minutes, stirring every few minutes until the onions are light brown. Add ginger and garlic, sauté for 2 more minutes.

3. Add tomato and spices, mix well, and cook covered on low heat for 5 minutes, stirring occasionally.

4. Mash tomatoes with the back of a spoon.

5. Add 1 cup water and garbanzo beans and mix well.

6. Bring to a boil over medium heat, and add salt.

7. Cover and cook for 20 minutes.

8. Use the back of a spoon to mash some of the garbanzo beans.

Add lemon juice, garnish with chopped cilantro, and serve with basmati rice and naan or roti.

🎵 PLAYLIST HIGHLIGHTS

Warm Up

Clocks – Coldplay

Lost Girls – Tilly and the Wall

Before-work Cardio

I only did two miles because I struggled with shin splints, especially on my left leg. I've had this problem off and on, but usually they let up after the first mile. Since I had to go more slowly, I ran out of time. I did six minutes on the arm bike maintaining 60 RPM and about 10 minutes on the mat, doing planks and leg and core work.

Flightless Bird, American Mouth – Iron & Wine

Happy Ending – MIKA

Dreams Be Dreams – Jack Johnson

Tore My Heart – OONA

The Con – Tegan and Sara

Count on Me – Bruno Mars (So wholesome)

Happy – Pharrell Williams (So sappy, but I love this song.)

Lovers' Eyes – Mumford and Sons (I set this one on repeat through arm bike—so great.)

Day 11, April 9, 2014

> *"Show me the buffet."*
> —John Pinette

I was surprised at how moved I was at seeing Su Meck at her book signing in Rockville. Su was on the talk show and book-signing circuit after her gripping memoir *I Forgot to Remember* was published. In the book, Su describes her survival and recovery from a devastating brain injury when her son Ben was a baby. I got to know Su when Ben and Mia performed in the "Laramie Project" together their senior year of high school. Su's daughter, Kassidy, did musical theater with Adin, and they were members of the same show choir. Su and I were stage moms and volunteers who drove our kids to rehearsals, collected props, and raised money for the youth theater group—Act Two Performing Arts before it became ActTwo@Levine—and threw cast parties for the kids.

Su had always been friendly and pleasant and enjoyed talking about her son Patrick, the diver, who had no interest in theater. We had met Patrick for the first time at the book signing, where Su told one of our friends that although she always carried a book with her to rehearsals back then, the brain injury had left her without the ability to read. She just wanted to fit in and seem normal. Su and her husband, who now live in Massachusetts, had made a decision to keep her injury a secret, and not one of the moms who socialized with Su had a clue until she told us about the book just before it was published.

Su's story is honest and touching. Woven throughout the pages of her memoir are the moments when she felt normal. There weren't many of these, but they formed the foundation of her survival. She said one thing she could count on were her gigs teaching aerobics or some other fitness class at a health club, probably what we would have called Equinox in the 80s, wearing our Jane Fonda leg warmers and leotards. There are disturbing moments as well, and it's hard not to feel like we all let Su down by enabling her to keep her struggle a secret. Her loneliness permeates the book, and I think we all feel a little guilty about that.

It was great to be together to catch up and to celebrate those moments of survival.

As we walked to our cars, my good friend Carmelita Watkinson suggested the two of us head to the bar at Seasons 52 for a late dinner. We had a great meal—I had a salad with sushi grade tuna, and both of us had a glass of Napa Valley Honig Sauvignon Blanc. In the center of the bar was Andy with the terrific voice at the piano. Andy is there every Tuesday night, and we're thinking we might be there too.

***

I was sad to read about the death of John Pinette at the age of fifty. Adin is the one who found the story and forwarded it to me. Apparently, the cause was a pulmonary embolism. When we lived in California and drove vast distances for practically any reason, Pinette's famous comedy special, *Show Me the Buffet*, was a favorite CD. He made fun of his size and his huffing and puffing around Disney World, and he recounted endlessly hilarious situations at the buffet.

In the end, not really that funny.

Very sad, Adin wrote.

***

Yesterday, I pushed myself to go to the gym for cardio before work and later had training with Adorable where we focused on my core, which I learned includes my lower back as well as my gut—duh—and my pecs, shoulders, and arms before heading to the book event. I did not have the same shin splint problem I had been having on Monday. Adorable had showed me some specific stretches to try before getting on the treadmill. It would be months and some guidance from my current physical therapist Dr. Kevin McGuinness before I was done with this problem, though.

🎵 PLAYLIST HIGHLIGHT

Only one is worth mentioning after such a long and full day.

Talk Dirty – Jason Derulo featuring 2 Chainz
(I've put this one in the same category as "Candy Shop" by 50 Cent. Seriously great stuff, but do we need to be exposed to this much explicit language? Jason Derulo?)

Day 12, April 10, 2014

> *"This is how I roll."*
> —LMFAO, "Sexy and I Know It"

It was probably only for a second, but I felt myself shrug when I stepped off the scale.

I'm fine just the way I am.

Adorable and I decided to put off getting me back on the scale, at least for this week.

"We can do that when you feel absolutely great," he said. Reuel is adorable, but he's also a genius.

This morning, I arrived at the gym a little earlier than usual. Because I knew I had training after work, I wanted to be more thoughtful about how much time I would spend on the treadmill, the arm bike, and maybe the recumbent bike, which my orthopedic surgeon had said would be good for my knees.

At 2.25 miles in, walking at a brisk 3.7 MPH, I decided I wanted more time on the arm bike, and I was feeling healthy—I had no issues with my shins, knees, or lower back, and I did not feel out of breath. It was during—of all songs—"Sexy and I Know It"—that I decided to increase my speed to 3.9 MPH and then 4.0 MPH, at which point the only way I could keep up was to start jogging.

I am not exaggerating when I tell you I fully expected my skeleton to begin crumbling to the floor.

I stayed with it, and there I was, running at a very acceptable pace for the next three quarters of a mile. No issues or problems—crazy! I started to crack up and nearly rolled off the back of the treadmill when I caught one of Adorable's clients I saw every morning out of the corner of my eye doing a double take as he was coming up from a bench press, not to mention the guy running next to me, who fed me a side-glance or two. Once I fell into a rhythm, I took a video selfie to ensure I was actually jogging and not simply thinking about jogging. I know I was listening to "No Church in the Wild" at that point because the music paused when the camera was recording, and I instantly thought, that's an Apple bug that needs a fix. Why can't the camera operate while the phone is playing music?

I did my five minutes on the arm bike, maintaining 60 RPM, but I never made it to the recumbent bike, since I forgot it. The last time I ran anywhere in sneakers and not heels catching a bus was between the bases during a high school softball game. What a sense of euphoria! It has been with me all day, and I can't wait to see where this takes me.

***

🎵 PLAYLIST HIGHLIGHTS

This was a great selection this morning, particularly in this order.

Switch – Will Smith

Don't Stop the Party – Pitbull (Adorable Shazamed this for me when it was playing in the training room during a set of straight-leg lifts a few nights ago. This is old, where've I been?)

Where Is the Love – Black Eyed Peas

My Humps – Black Eyed Peas (Always makes me smile, especially when I remember my niece singing this one from her booster seat in my car.)

We Be Burning – Sean Paul

Lose Yourself – Eminem (Nearly bought a Chrysler because of how great this song is.)

Dry Your Eyes – The Streets

Temperature – Sean Paul

The Boogie That Be – Black Eyed Peas (Kind of heavy on Fergie this morning.)

Club Can't Handle Me – Flo Rida

Hard Knock Life (Ghetto Version) – Jay Z (I'm a huge fan and loved his memoir.)

Sexy and I Know It – LMFAO (I know, I know.)

Stronger – Kanye

Touch the Sky – Kanye and Lupe Fiasco

No Church in the Wild – Kanye and Jay Z

Sunshine – Mos Def

Crazy Kids – Kesha

The Way I Are – Timbaland

Hey Ya! – OutKast

Day 20, April 18, 2014

> *"La drogue agit sur moi lentement."*
> —Yelle, "Comme Un Enfant"

Here is the thing about endorphins: OMG they are for real.

Yesterday I had lunch with my colleague Jill, and in the cab back to the office, I had landed in her lap as her foot and bottom wedged under the front passenger seat and on the floor of the taxi. Neither of us was wearing a seat belt, as we had been deep in conversation from the time we hailed the cab until the moment it suddenly stopped within inches of plowing into a car that was trying to sneak a left turn. I saw the other car—if the cab driver had not slammed on the brakes at that very moment, we would have been sitting on that driver's lap.

Jill's ankle hurt, but she was okay walking back into our building. Later that evening as I was riding to the garage in the elevator, two other colleagues commented that I seemed to be okay after the accident in the cab.

"Is Jill okay?"

"She's limping pretty badly and probably going to the ER tonight."

Really?

I started to tell them what had happened, but when I described sitting on Jill's lap on the floor of the cab, I burst into the most ridiculous and uncontrollably hysterical laughter. One of the other colleagues smiled, too, but more in reaction to my face than to the situation, which was not funny. We had almost had a car accident, and now Jill, who's about to take leave and have down time with her family for Easter, was headed to the emergency room.

I'm chuckling right now as I'm writing this. It's like I'm high on morphine. And, yes, I know what that's like, because I delivered Mia in a Philadelphia city hospital while the patient in the room next to mine coded and died of preeclampsia. There was so much chaos in and around my hospital room, with men and women in white coats and scrubs racing around, trying to forget about me, that for a minute I imagined I was in an episode of *St. Elsewhere*. No one was available to perform an epidural, so the resident decided morphine would put everything on pause. I don't remember a lot about my labor experiences with either of my children, but I do remember the morphine that day.

Apparently, endorphins are considered endogenous morphine. And I think the effect must be cumulative, because as I'm adding running to my daily cardio and upping my speed a bit, I am seriously high all day. I can barely keep a straight face, even in a training session with Adorable when my shoulders are obviously on fire.

I just can't help myself.

He's watching me, concentrating deeply.

And I'm cracking up.

Do people talk about this? Maybe I'm just particularly sensitive and the effect is exaggerated, but I have a serious job and a lot of work to do, and this is more than a feeling of well-being.

***

It has been two weeks since I last weighed in at the gym, and in discussing whether I should do it tonight, both Lord Baltimore and Mia pointed out the good and the bad. Neither wanted to persuade me to weigh myself, because they were worried I'd be discouraged if I hadn't lost any weight. But then they didn't want to dissuade me, either. They didn't want it to seem as if they thought I looked like I hadn't lost any weight.

It's fine.

I had lost one pound, which does not even seem remotely possible considering what I've been doing to my body and not putting into my body. The numbers are at least moving in the right direction, and I feel good. Whoever said life is good must have been high on endorphins.

Life is good.

***

During a training session last week, I asked Adorable what we were working when it felt as if we were strengthening my chest muscles, which on a scale of 1 to 10 did not seem to be a top problem spot.

"The pectoral muscles."

"Why?"

"Working the pecs is clutch."

"Clutch?"

"The pec's a really big muscle and working big muscles helps you burn calories."

"Clutch?"

"The larger muscle groups are *clutch* in terms of burning more calories."

I've been trying to use "clutch" in a sentence all day, but the best I can do is, "I really like the Cubist *minaudière* clutch bag on the J. Crew website."

***

I did two long road trips last weekend, and for at least three hours I had Adin in the car with me while I was driving him back to school. We talked about music for a good chunk of the time. Both he and Mia have always been up on the latest music trends, but Adin in particular, both because he has been a dancer/choreographer since he was in middle school and because he has a knack for discovering music that is especially right for movement, so that's why I get a lot of ideas from him. This time, he turned me on to "Comme Un Enfant" from the French band Yelle's album *Safari Disco Club*. He's still confounded by my lack of enthusiasm for Beyoncé, even if I'm president of the Jay Z fan club.

"She's all about empowering women, Mom, you should love her."

"I've got endorphins, honey. I'd be lethal if I had any more empowerment."

Day 23, April 21, 2014

> *"Everybody's looking for something"*
> —Eurythmics, "Sweet Dreams"

A Motown classic washed over the final scene of August Wilson's *Two Trains Running,* which I saw at Round House Theatre in Bethesda. But after three hours of so much dialogue, I almost expected to hear Vangelis' "Chariots of Fire" as the actors took their well-deserved bows. The story is set in Pittsburgh's Hill District overlooking downtown Pittsburgh at the end of the Hill's heyday in 1969 Everything on stage happens in a diner owned by Memphis, the play's central character, but it was Risa who had caught my attention.

Lord Baltimore and I went to the play with my good friend Mimi Kress and her husband, photographer Michael Kress. Mimi works as many long hours as any woman I know, but there she is nearly every morning, at the gym by 6:00 a.m. She's got that *je ne sais quoi* that I've started to recognize in women of my age who have figured out what works for them. During intermission, Mimi and I realized Lord Baltimore and Michael had not noticed the deep scars deforming Risa's legs when she had crossed the stage as the diner's waitress.

How could they miss that?

This was the first thing Mimi and I noticed when we met Risa, a gorgeous woman—beautifully played at Round House by Shannon Dorsey—who had used a blade to cut her legs as a girl to avoid the unwanted attention of men. There was some backstory here that Wilson didn't get into, but we got the point that the males in Risa's life were all about asking her for something, especially Memphis, her boss.

So, when the likable Sterling finally comes out with it and lets Risa know how he feels about her—despite her "ugly" legs—Risa gives herself a little push and confronts her own desires. It's a poignant moment in the play—if underplayed in the Round House version—and although Wilson doesn't typically write a lot of female characters, he got this one right. I found it interesting that the two males we were with in the audience never saw the scars until Sterling mentioned them. In that way, Lord Baltimore and Michael were kind of like Sterling, who looked at Risa's legs but never paid them any attention. Even as I am determined to lose weight and sport sleeveless blouses with First Lady ease, I am still marveling at how much I am responsible not only for my own self-image but also for the image others have of me.

On the way home from dinner in Baltimore last night, I listened to Muddy Waters's soulful "Still a Fool," which is where the title of the play comes from, and I thought about the word "journey" and how often this word as a concept is simply inadequate.

There's two trains running

Well ain't nary one—ho!—going my way

***

I feel so much better about everything. I'm not only pulling myself up into a side plank, I am holding a side plank, even on my right side. I've been practicing yoga for several years, yet I've always been bothered by how difficult the down dog position is for me because of the weakness in my right wrist, which I broke years ago. To use Adorable's word, holding up my core with my right arm is nothing short of *epic*.

A side effect is that I am also starting to feel impatient for a ripped abdomen, even though I'm a long way off—if ever—from anything even close to that. I'm almost a little embarrassed to admit this.

I've changed my attitudes about fitness and daydream about being fit.

And smokin'.

🎵 PLAYLIST HIGHLIGHTS

2-hour workouts Saturday and Sunday morning (1 hour cardio / 3 miles total / 2 miles at 4.2 MPH (!) / 6 minutes on the arm bike maintaining 70 RPM / 1 hour on the mat and cool arm and leg stretches Adorable showed me)

Sunshine – Rye Rye

Don't Stop the Party – Pitbull

Quiet Dog – Mos Def

Comme Un Enfant – Yelle

212 – Azealia Banks

Pump It – Black Eyed Peas

After Party – Keith Milgaten/ Keith Stanfield

Right Round – Flo Rida (My happy place.)

Envy – 116

m.A.A.d city – Kendrick Lamar

In da Club – 50 Cent

Don't Matter – Akon

Land – Patti Smith

Sweet Dreams – Eurythmics (I like the remix.)

Everyone's the Same – Alice Anna (My sister-in-law Lindsey's husband, Scott Smith, played guitar in this Baltimore band.)

Happy – Pharrell Williams

Lovers' Eyes – Mumford and Sons

Day 25, April 23, 2014

"I am the luckiest."
—Ben Folds, "The Luckiest"

Last week the *New York Times* ran a story about gyms using personal fitness devices to track clients' activity. Basically, clients buy some sort of wearable activity tracker that allows their trainer to monitor their every move. So, for example, if I told Adorable that this morning I ran 2 miles at 4.2 MPH, Adorable could either say he already knew that or that it was more like 1.5 miles, because he's got my activity data on his phone.

When I asked Adorable about this, he didn't seem all that engaged one way or the other.

I think that's because he knew he probably wouldn't need an electronic device to monitor his clients' data. I push myself simply by knowing he's in the building when I'm running on the treadmill. I'm sure I'd be walking up and down nine flights of stairs to get to and from my office if I knew he was carrying my physical activity data in his pocket.

I want to take back the comment I made earlier about motivation. Adorable had told me that many clients (not only his) rely on their trainers to motivate them (think drill sergeant). I had considered that idea but concluded I am the only person who can motivate me.

Not.

Obviously, I am motivated to get results, but I do not (yet) have the ability to push myself to get there. I've completely crossed over and bought in to the whole trainer vibe. I need this. I need to be pushed. Someone with skill needs to tell me how high and how long and how far. It's not in my nature to go much beyond what my brain signals is safe.

And I don't get that endorphin rush unless I push myself harder than I thought possible. It's the sprinting, going harder and longer at whatever, that gives me the happy pill.

I need this.

**

A few weeks ago, Adorable had me do repetitions on the horrible back extension machine, and then immediately "flex" my stomach on the machine next to it without a break. He calls that a "super set," and I've tried to duplicate the super set concept when I go from the treadmill (without a cool down) to the arm bike to holding a plank in the mornings before work. I benefit from taking breaks in between sets or from a cool down after running, but I get the point of the super set. It's another way to get that unexpected fast rush.

Flex my stomach? If you can visualize that, let me know.

We got on the subject of the super set tonight because we were talking about endurance and how to boost it. For my morning workouts, Adorable suggested I try ramping up my speed on the treadmill for 30 seconds, and then taking it back down, and to do this throughout my three miles.

***

The millennial on the treadmill next to me was furiously texting while running a nine-minute mile. I was worried she might step over the edge, but she was completely in control.

Later that evening in my kitchen, I was having difficulty texting Mia, who was on a quiet bus from Boston back to New York, while eating a piece of matzah.

***

Yesterday morning I had to take my car in for service because it had two flat tires. Both tires were punctured with nails, so I assumed I must have driven into a construction zone. Later, in the shower, I winced when I put my foot down at a certain angle and thought maybe I had bruised something. I took a look and saw I had a splinter deep in the sole of my right foot.

As a girl from the beaches of Long Island who has had a lot of experience with splinters, I typically leave them and let them rise to the surface on their own. But this morning I thought I'd try to get it out so I wouldn't have any problems running. I took out my tweezer kit (everyone has one, right?) and used the sharpest tool to pry out the small piece of wood. After some time, I pulled it out in one piece and took a look at it. It was sharp, like a nail.

Is it just me, or is someone using a voodoo doll to cast a spell on me?

Before-work Cardio

(3 miles total/ 2 miles at 4.2 MPH / 5 minutes on the arm bike maintaining 70 RPM / arm stretches)

🎵 **PLAYLIST HIGHLIGHTS**

Mellow this morning as I was fairly sleep-deprived.

What a Piece of Work Is Man – From the soundtrack of the Broadway musical *Hair*

After Party – Keith Milgaten and Keith Stanfield

Hey Baby – Pitbull

When a Man Loves a Woman – Aaron Neville

Count on Me – Bruno Mars

Paperweight – Joshua Radin and Schuyler Fisk

Waiting on the World to Change – John Mayer

Mad World – from Donnie Darko

Clocks – Coldplay

Tiny Dancer – Ben Folds cover (Such an amazing pianist.)

The Luckiest – Ben Folds

Day 29, April 27, 2014

> *"Then I realized I was swimming."*
> —Florence + the Machine, "Swimming"

You have to be smart about your addictions.

I warmed up for 30 minutes on the treadmill, including a 1-mile run, early on Friday before my morning training session and followed Adorable's suggestion to include a minute of sprinting sprinkled in two or three times during my run.

During training, I had a lot of discomfort in my calves and my left shin, and by the end of the hour, Adorable suggested I take the weekend off from running, or even walking, on the treadmill.

"Okay."

But okay was not what I was thinking. I doubted I could get through the next two days without this.

I told Adorable I'd swim.

"Nice."

Nearly everyone I knew growing up on Long Island was a swimmer. Even as adults, my father, Len, and my sisters Sherry, Phyllis, and Ilene, swim regularly, and I swam in the Johns Hopkins University pool when I was in graduate school. Once I started dying my hair, though, getting my head soaked in a tank of chlorine lost its appeal for me. I hadn't even glanced at the Equinox pool, which by the way was salt water, so I didn't know what to expect when I showed up on Saturday morning.

But before I could swim in the pool, I needed to stop at a sporting goods store to pick up a silicone swim cap, goggles from this decade, and a racing suit, because I was sure my

Karla Colletto was never meant to get wet. City Sports fit me in a cap that would work for my head and hair and goggles with the correct "orbit" for my face. I picked the cheapest suit on the rack that didn't look too much like I knew what I was doing. They had "swim paddles" for your hands that added resistance to your work out, but I knew enough to talk to Adorable first before investing in a pair of lobster claws.

I put the suit on in the locker room and worked carefully to tuck each strand of hair into the cap. Since City Sports had already sized the goggles for me, all I needed to do was set them on my face, walk into the pool area, and get into the water. But as I was about to step onto the ladder, a trainer working with a client in the pool (the client was in the pool; the trainer was walking on the deck as she swam) greeted me in that very sincere friendly way that made me want to lift the cap off my ears so I could return the pleasantry. I settled everything back into the cap and onto my face and got in the water, sharing a lane with Mark Spitz.

After two lengths, Spitz was waiting for me, and he politely suggested that since there were only the two of us in the lane, he could take the rope and I could take the outside.

"If someone else comes, we can swim in a circle."

I was good with that but had to lift the cap off my ears to hear him and the goggles off my face to see him, so I was still adjusting everything when he returned from another two lengths.

"How do you keep track of how many lengths you're doing?"

"I don't, I just know that it takes me fifty seconds to do two lengths."

He wasn't wearing a watch. "How do you know it's fifty seconds?"

He pointed behind my head. I turned around and saw the practically life-size stopwatch sitting on the edge of the pool.

"Ahh."

I kept track of my time. I was varying between 70 and 80 seconds for two 25-meter lengths. I was never sure whether I was swimming 70 or 80 seconds or 70 or 80 seconds plus 60 seconds because I only saw the stopwatch twice during my sprint—once when I started and once when I finished.

(By Sunday, when I was more acclimated to the pool and the whole swimming culture, I figured out that I was actually taking 70 or 80 seconds per two lengths, so that was good information. I was resting about 20 seconds after every two lengths, but I was already pushing myself, so there was no getting around that.)

After the nausea passed and I realized I had been swimming close to an hour, I started to worry that I'd be there all day, because I knew I wasn't getting out of the water before Spitz. It had been months since my last bikini wax, and I hadn't been able to get an appointment until later in the afternoon. Thankfully, after about 55 minutes, he stepped out of the water onto the side of the deck and started to towel off, waiting for me at the end to tell me to have a nice day. I used some of his mojo and pumped it up for the last 10 minutes.

And yes, it stayed with me the rest of the day.

At a birthday dinner for my mother on Sunday night, I asked Ilene about the swim cap thing, because my hair was soaked even though the cap fit snugly on my head.

"None of them work."

"You're an engineer and dad's a patent attorney, and NASA can put a man on the moon. We can't get a cap that keeps our hair dry?"

"Yeah, I know."

"What about that vacuum sealed bag that Isaac and Adin wore in the shower recovering from their knee and ankle surgeries? Why can't we wear that over our hair?"

I caught my nephew Isaac cracking a smile, but I seriously wanted to add swimming to my regimen. My workout in the pool gave me an endorphin-induced high that fed my addiction. But Len had had green hair for years, and I was paying a lot of money to get the Brazilian Keratin treatment every five or six months. I ordered the All Star Bubble Cap from Aqua Gear, but since it only cost $7.83, I didn't have high hopes.

Ilene swims with a watch that keeps track of her distance, and she said she always does at least 32 laps—a mile.

I told her Triathlete had suggested I get the waterproof iPod shuffle from Waterfi.

"Don't you just want to let your mind wander while you swim, think about recipes, maybe listen to the sound of the water?"

My sister knows me, and, well, I did think about recipes during my swim this morning, as well as what I *would* be listening to if I were listening to music. And I had made Tamara's ratatouille from Ottolenghi's *Plenty* and quinoa with dried cherries and pistachios this afternoon.

"Research—and not just Adin's middle school science project—shows that there's a physiological chain reaction to music and rhythm that enhances athletic performance," I said.

Though she heard me out while loading the dishwasher, Ilene wasn't buying it. Her husband Ethan, though, had been talking about getting a waterproof iPod for years.

"Let me know what you think," he glanced at my sister before turning to me. "Maybe it'll make a good Father's Day present."

Will do.

CHAPTER 2 –
WHY YOU NEED A
STRATEGY

Day 39, May 7, 2014

> *"Work it, make it, do it."*
> —Daft Punk, "Harder, Better, Faster, Stronger"

From what I'm reading, I might be the only woman who wears underwear with her Lululemons, but here I am. I did not enjoy my forced day off from working out on Monday. I was cranky and lethargic. If it weren't for my lovely Vassar friend Liz Nagy, who took me out to see the always funny Leslie Mann in *The Other Woman* after work, I'm sure I would have found Adin's exercise mat and held a few planks.

Then I would have had to tell Adorable and Triathlete and Wonderful. It was the first thing Adorable asked me at our morning training.

"Yes, I took yesterday off."

"You feel good? Muscles rested?"

"Whatever."

How unexpected is it that just a month ago I existed blissfully in an anti-exercise bubble so removed from fitness culture? I don't want to be that person who goes on and on about how you should eat this or exercise like that, but I've kind of turned into her.

Here's why.

More than 2,300 people participated in Saturday's 5K to raise funds for the Robert Packard Center for ALS Research in Baltimore. Our team—formed a year after my father-in-law's death—was small compared to the teams of twenty or more people wearing the names of loved ones on their shirts and banners. We walked and talked, mostly about the mix of quirky gourmet restaurants and bars lining the streets of Fells Point and Canton, and we lingered over a decadent breakfast together after the race at Miss Shirley's Café. Even though it was a sad day remembering our family's loss, it was a happy and chatty group around the table, including Lord Baltimore, my parents, Harriet and Len; Mia; Roland's widow and Lord Baltimore's stepmother, Vada Walker; and Lord Baltimore's sisters Hope, Nicole, and Lindsey.

I'd supported my friends' and my friends' children participating in fitness fundraising events, so how is it that this was my first one? And it wasn't that I'd been unaware of the popularity of fitness charity events. In 2007, I had written about how charity walks not only raise millions of dollars, but they also increase awareness about the importance of physical fitness.

For context on how out of step I've been, according to statistics collected by the Run Walk Ride Fundraising Council, in 2012, 11.9 million people participated in 35,000 run/walk charity fundraising events, raising a whopping $1.68 billion. There is an incredible community commitment to these events. I showed up with my water bottle and my banana, but I didn't need either. There were corporate sponsors and vendors donating crates full of bananas, water, and energy bars. Musicians performed on stages in the middle of it all, and Baltimore's finest police officers blocked off the race route and held traffic back for us as we strolled along.

I asked my sister Ilene if she'd ever done one of these walks.

"A million."

"Really?" She'd never asked me for a donation.

"I always do the autism and brain cancer races. I don't ask people to donate, as I usually donate myself."

I have no idea what I used to do with my time. Or money.

***

I'm a month and a half into training, and I've finally figured out that getting stronger does not make future sessions easier. Somehow, I thought it would, because this is intuitive and the concept behind practice, practice, practice. Just as I become able to hold a side plank or not get emotional on that horrible back machine, Adorable finds some other way to turn it up.

As in holding a plank for three minutes while balancing your feet on a Bosu ball, AND THEN holding a plank while balancing your feet on a Bosu ball and alternating lifting your legs from the hip flexors, AND THEN super setting the whole thing.

He says not hitting a plateau is kind of the point of training. I get that. I just thought it wouldn't be so *uncomfortable*. Adorable, like many trainers, is proficient at reading nonverbal cues, and he's starting to tell me where I am before I ask him. As this gets more challenging, I need to know how much longer or how much more so I can mentally focus on the "okay, you're done." This is a new development, and I hope it means I'll start seeing some results, especially in my arms and back.

Lord Baltimore commented over the weekend that he thinks I look like I'm "sculpting." I'm not seeing that yet, but if he is, that works for me.

***

It felt so great to run yesterday morning before training, but Adorable recommended I skip the treadmill for the rest of this week and get back in the pool.

I swam for 45 minutes this morning, but with about a 20-second break after every two lengths, which I noticed is what most people do. And that's not because everyone is exhausted after two lengths; it's because the swim sportswear industry has not kept up with the standards set by the running, or even yoga, industry. Before I get in the pool, I've got my waterproof ear buds tucked under my silicone cap and my fitted goggles placed on my face. After two lengths, the sides of the cap have slipped up, exposing my ears and the buds, and the front of the cap has slipped down, pressing into my goggles, which by now have suctioned themselves deeply into the skin under my eyes.

Every time I look up, there's a person readjusting something by the side of the pool.

I've given up trying to keep my hair dry. Although Adelia Varga, the genius Brazilian hairstylist who does my keratin straightening treatment, told me I'm okay swimming in a salt water pool even if I'm supposed to avoid products with sodium chloride, I'm reluctantly beginning to accept the fact that I might need to embrace my naturally curly, frizzy hair, at least for a while. So far the color is holding, but it's still early.

***

I took a core yoga flow class on Tuesday night. I've never seen the yoga studio so crowded. Just when you thought the room was completely full, five people would walk in and the teacher would settle them into the tiniest spots. Our mats were practically touching. I used to attend this six o'clock morning class, and while others joined Equinox for the chilled, eucalyptus-soaked towels, I had joined for the early morning yoga class. It was so nice to take the evening class.

Everything we're doing tonight is about creating space... creating space for the breath...

Before-work cardio

In the pool.

(45 minutes total—2 lengths at 70 seconds)

🎵 PLAYLIST HIGHLIGHTS

Nothing like hip-hop before the sun rises.

Stronger – Kanye West

212 – Azealia Banks

Talk Dirty – Jason Derulo

Don't Stop the Party – Pitbull

Quiet Dog – Mos Def

Comme Un Enfant – Yelle

We Run the Night – Havana Brown (I put this one on repeat.)

Hey Baby – Pitbull

The Light – Common

Blind – Kesha

Burn – Meek Mill

Freestyle – Bassnectar

Turn Down for What – DJ Snake and Lil Jon

Gin and Juice – Snoop Dog

After Party – Keith Milgaten and Keith Stanfield

Day 44, May 12, 2014

> *"I live for little moments."*
> —Brad Paisley, "Little Moments"

The last time I had attended a college reunion, it was such a long drive to Vassar that the first thing I did when I arrived on campus was find an open building with a bathroom. When I came out of the stall, there was quite a crowd in there. I looked around for someone I knew and saw a woman wearing a tag with my year on it, and I thought, *she must be the mother of a classmate.*

Walking out to my car in the parking lot, a (dim) light bulb went off.

She *is* a classmate.

I am a month away from my reunion, and both Ripped and I intend to arrive at Vassar looking good. We ran into each other last week after her training session with Adorable. A single hug, and I could tell she is a woman on a mission. It's crunch time.

The scale has not been my friend these last few weeks, but on Friday I came across a pair of jeans hanging in my closet that I remembered wearing in Florida to celebrate my parents' fiftieth wedding anniversary ten years ago. I put them on, and they fit—not great, but passably. I tried them on again on Saturday and Sunday to be sure. I mentioned this to Lord Baltimore, mostly because they are the greatest jeans.

"You have pants in your closet from ten years ago?"

Like most women, I have an area of my closet sectioned off for special things I never wear. I am not a sentimental person, so only a few items have real significance, and only a handful still have the tags. My Laura Ashley cotton wedding dress is there—I looked like a dairy maid at my wedding, but when Halloween came around that year, I rocked Glinda from the *Wizard of Oz* in that dress. I must have been very slim at my nephew Sam Walker's bar mitzvah, because that gorgeous sleeveless black velvet dress looks tiny, and I probably should have given it away years ago.

***

I'm doing workarounds with my workouts because (a) I need to stay out of the pool for a week because I'm giving the Brazilian Keratin treatment one last try, and I just had it done; and (b) my left knee started to ache after sprints on the treadmill on Thursday night.

I met with my orthopedic surgeon on Friday, and he suggested (for the millionth time) that I use the recumbent bike to strengthen the muscles in and around my knees.

As boring as that machine is, I can feel the benefit. Both Saturday (50 minutes—that was before I had a chance to check in with Adorable, who suggested 20 to 30 minutes or three miles) and Sunday I used the recumbent bike first, and then did six minutes on the arm bike maintaining 70 RPM, and then went to the mat for some floor work. This morning I made sure to do some core work that includes my back because I've got a training session tomorrow morning, and I've noticed that whenever I poop out it's usually because of my back. If I have time on Wednesday morning, my plan is to do the recumbent bike, the arm bike, and then walk on the treadmill at a brisk pace for three miles.

I tried to read my next book club book on the bike on Saturday, but after a few pages of *Devil in a Blue Dress*, I realized if I were on the trail on my Jamis Allegro, I would be meandering at a very annoying pace. I'm still not able to watch or read anything while I'm working out—it requires my full attention. My self-imposed weigh-in is on Thursday night. I know it's not about the weight, but I might cry this time if I don't see the numbers moving down, so whether I'm training or pumping my legs or arms on any kind of machine, I'm doing it full-out.

Naturally I'm continuing to try to be smart about what I eat and when. I went with Ilene to a "Metabolism Re-Start" workshop at EB Nutrition in Rockville last Thursday night, and amid registered dietician Elizabeth Blumberg's dense PowerPoint slides, I came away with a few kernels of wisdom:

◊ "Metabolism" is the chemical process that occurs within an organism to maintain life. So essentially your metabolism is responsible for ensuring that all processes in your body are carried out efficiently. Maybe you knew this, but for me, it's cool to think about my metabolism as the CEO of my body.

◊ Sugar is the enemy. Among other effects, when you experience stress, the body releases a stress hormone called cortisol, which triggers a release of sugar and fat into the bloodstream. Elizabeth said basically stress is like going through the Dairy Queen drive-through. Although I didn't completely get the analogy, I did wonder whether there was a Dairy Queen nearby.

◊ A slow metabolism can be caused by emotional toxicity. Stored conscious or subconscious beliefs and thought patterns contribute to emotional toxicity. I'm still processing this one.

Elizabeth does not approve of my freshly squeezed orange juice and banana before morning workouts because they have too much sugar. I've asked around, and a lot of people don't eat anything before their morning workout. I've never tried that, but I did try cutting out the OJ and having a piece of toast instead of the banana before a morning training session with Adorable, and I lost both my focus and my energy, which I imagine was as disappointing for him as it was for me.

I know the OJ and the banana have a lot of sugar, but isn't that the point? I could literally skip down East-West Highway to get to the gym in the mornings. The combination is like a hypodermic shot in the arm that gets me through the toughest training or the most rigorous cardio workout.

I liked Elizabeth, and if I had an hour to spare and I was considering seeing a nutritionist, I'd see her, but we'd have to agree to disagree on this point for now.

***

Today was Day 1 of Triathlete's training for her race in August. I sent her a cheery rise and shine text at 5:30 this morning, and in return she brought us the most delicious lunch: Kale and Quinoa Salad with Ricotta Salata from Smitten Kitchen—she substituted feta for the ricotta, which was perfect.

***

When my colleague and friend Beth Cooper asked me about my Mothers' Day, I told her I had missed seeing Mia and Adin but was impressed and touched that they'd conspired to send me a fabulous Manduko yoga bag, which arrived via Amazon on Saturday.

"Whose idea do you think it was?"

"Sounds like a trick question," I said. "But when Mia visited last weekend, she gave me a quick, concerned look after she noticed I was dragging my workout gear around in my Longchamp."

***

I was sad my BFF Carmelita Watkinson was unable to join me tonight for Chris's yin yoga class. She had strained her back gardening that afternoon and needed to rest.

I think Chris would have been happy Carm spent the sunny day in her garden.

"See if you can find the space between your thoughts," Chris said. "If you can get comfortable, see if you can flourish there."

For those of us who could stay, Chris led us through an extra-long *savasana,* which was our reward for our hard work holding poses for up to five minutes.

"There isn't a more important personal relationship than the one we're having here right now with ourselves."

Love this guru.

🎵 PLAYLIST HIGHLIGHTS

My father had surprised me when he told me he's a country music fan—I had no idea! Here's some of what I put on his iPod and enjoyed during my workouts over the weekend:

Need You Now – Antebellum

Storyline – Hunter Hayes

Play It Again –Luke Bryan

Wild Card – Hunter Hayes

Wheels of Love – Emmylou Harris

This Is Country Music – Brad Paisley

Little Moments – Brad Paisley (Love this one.)

Born Country – Alabama

Rewind – Rascal Flatts

Boys 'Round Here – Blake Shelton

On the Road Again – Willie Nelson (Of course.)

Always on My Mind – Willie Nelson

Ring of Fire – Johnny Cash

Folsom Prison Blues – Johnny Cash

Here Comes the Sun – Beatles (LOVE version)

While My Guitar Gently Weeps – Beatles (LOVE version)

Happy – Pharrell Williams

Brave – Sara Bareilles

Day 50, May 18, 2014

> *"I should probably warn you I'll be just fine."*
> —Pharrell Williams, "Happy"

As of Friday, I've lost four pounds since Day 1. That's 3.31 percent of my body weight and a loss of three pounds in two weeks.

"You're a teeny tiny person," Lord Baltimore told me. "If you'd weighed three hundred pounds, at that rate, you would have lost nine pounds." I don't think that sounds very impressive, but I give him an A for effort.

I was on the Woodway treadmill in the middle of my training on Thursday when I realized I had forgotten to get on the scale. For someone who was keenly focused on losing 20 pounds by the end of this thing, it was crazy that I had let it slip my mind. Earlier in the week, Adorable might have been trying to make me feel better when he told me I had crossed another barrier after a nearly complete meltdown during incredibly challenging core work, but I think he's right. I'm on the other side of my obsession with the scale.

Still, when I weighed in at 117 at my doctor's office on Friday, I cracked a small smile. It has been eight weeks, and I feel better, my clothes fit better, I've got much more energy, and I crave physical activity.

Now when I think about food, I think about fuel. I'm eating what I need instead of what I want, and that's a big shift for me. Cooking in my own kitchen and eating out in restaurants are still important aspects of my social life, and when we were at dinner on Saturday night at Black's Bar and Kitchen in Bethesda with Vassar friends, including Ellen Radish and her husband, Seth Zarny, who's been a runner since college, I built a meal around what I had done earlier in the day.

Black's is an easy place to do this, because the food is so good at every course that you can piece together just the right mix of vegetables, protein, and complex carbs with little effort. For appetizers, we shared oysters and bruschetta with white beans and prosciutto. For my entree, I had salad greens with avocado and grilled shrimp and a side of grilled cauliflower. I worried about ordering a salad for dinner, but nobody seemed to notice or care. It was what I needed, because earlier, after my two-hour workout on my own at Equinox, I had already eaten more than enough protein and complex carbs for the day.

Elizabeth, the nutritionist from the workshop I went to a few weeks ago, had advised against eating sugar—including fruit or wine—within three hours of bedtime. Since our reservation was on the early side, I had two small (3 oz.) glasses of wine with dinner and the homemade guava and passion fruit sorbet for dessert. After a few spoonfuls, I passed the bowl around the table.

(By the way, celebrity sighting at Black's: then National Security Advisor Susan Rice was having dinner with her husband at the table next to ours.)

***

My internist is monitoring my high blood pressure. For starters, he told me to go off ibuprofen cold turkey, starting immediately. I've been on a daily dose of ibuprofen for osteoarthritis symptoms for as long as I can remember, which is at least a decade. He told me to switch to acetaminophen and gave me a referral to see a rheumatologist in July. I didn't have any Tylenol in the house and didn't pick any up until early Sunday morning, when I woke up feeling ancient. I took the extra-strength extended release tablets (didn't even know they made these), and I feel okay. We'll see.

***

After a very productive session with Adorable this morning focusing on increasing my stamina and strengthening the muscles in my core, Lord Baltimore and I took out our bikes for the first time this year and picked up the Capital Crescent Trail from our path off Connecticut Avenue.

"I can see the benefit of working out twice a day," Lord Baltimore commented.

Yeah, me too.

***

At Adorable's suggestion, I'm on the recumbent bike for three miles at the beginning of working out or training, and for 10 minutes at the end. I'm seeing my orthopedist tomorrow morning to check out my left knee, which feels wonky from time to time, but I've seen a great improvement since I started using that bike.

🎵 PLAYLIST HIGHLIGHTS

Adin's been sending me some ideas—some new and some classic. I'll call this my Happy Mix.

Fancy – Iggy Azalea

Silver Screen (Shower Scene) – Felix Da Housecat

Feel Good – Gorillaz

Ball – by T.I. (Okay, maybe I should take this one off my happy mix.)

Happy Ending – Mika

Fly or Die – Rock Mafia

Hopeless Wanderer – Mumford and Sons

Where to Land – Travis Garland

Fast Car – Tracy Chapman

Do What You Want – Lady Gaga

Can't Hold Us – Macklemore and Ryan Lewis

Switch – Will Smith

Love the Way You Lie – Eminem

Where'd You Go – Fort Minor

Where Is the Love – Black Eyed Peas

Dry Your Eyes – The Streets

Ain't No Sunshine – Lighthouse Family

Reflektor – Arcade Fire

Pump It – Black Eyed Peas

Happy – Pharrell Williams (Corny, I know—but it gets me where I need to go.)

Rhythm of Love – Plain White T's

Day 58, May 26, 2014

> *"Sway to the rhythm of love."*
> —Plain White Ts, "Rhythm of Love"

All it takes is one patriotic holiday weekend to undo weeks of discipline and training: too much food, too much alcohol, too much sun, too much too much. There is no such thing as watching anything except watching everyone have fun, when you're in the Poconos for the first time in sixteen years with seventy-two members of your family, including many of the cousins you surrounded yourself with through most of your childhood in New York.

If my eight weeks of training and paying close attention to my diet has done anything for me, it's given me the stamina to party with the big boys.

I had such good intentions.

On Friday, I had an early morning training session with Adorable before fitting into a favorite pair of cutoffs and packing lunch for the long drive to Pennsylvania. On Saturday, I started the morning with a run on the treadmill and joined my cousins for Zumba, but somehow lost my way by lunchtime. (BTW, I was utterly uncoordinated at Zumba, which was disappointing, because I was super good at Jane Fonda's aerobics videos in the 1980s and even took her class in Beverly Hills wearing a shiny lime green leotard, light blue tights, and yellow leggings. Mia shot film of the Zumba class, but fortunately she used my iPhone, so I own the footage.)

Instead, during the weekend I alternated my High-Intensity Interval Training (bursts of intense hugging, drinking, and fast conversation and slowed down recovery periods of lounging by the pool and meandering remembrances around the fire pit) with low-intensity steady-state cardio (socializing at a lower intensity but maintaining it for extended periods from breakfast to lunch, to happy hour to dinner, to late night cocktails in the sports bar).

"Enough already with the Belkin stories," my cousin's wife said. "You're not the Kennedys." I had almost forgotten that her husband, my cousin, had visited me at Vassar so he could date a Vassar girl, which he did.

From the youngest cousin to my father, the family elder, all of us appeared remarkably blessed with health. I noticed this even as all of us had a little too much of everything. My eight-year-old cousin Marley blogs about the best / worst chicken fingers; my cousin Donna Nadler loads workouts, including yoga, onto her iPad, which she pulled out of her bag and hooked up to the resort's speakers when the yoga teacher didn't show up for Sunday's yoga class. And my niece Sofie's movement/meditation workshop incorporated movement into meditation to make it more comfortable, especially for people who have difficulty sitting for long periods of time. She's got a family full of followers.

I'm sure I'm not the only cousin slightly overwhelmed about how to get back on track and feeling worried about fitting into those workout pants, even the stretched-out ones, tomorrow morning. I wish I had been able to stay focused during a mere three days of distractions. I'm counting on a silver lining here that maybe I'll be motivated to push harder this week.

Tomorrow I'm adding serious rap to my playlist. I'm not going light this week. No happy mix starting tomorrow.

***

Bathed in the safety and security of my extended family, I read about the shooting in Santa Barbara over the weekend. The nightmarish visuals of menace juxtaposed with images of beauty haunt me. We have to fix this.

Day 65, June 2, 2014

> *"Slow down the time."*
> —Bon Iver, "Woods"

I always have the same feeling of embarrassment when I walk up the two flights of stairs and enter the main training floor of the gym huffing and puffing. Nevertheless, as I approach the row of treadmills or bikes, I instinctively settle on the one next to a gym goer. And I'm not the only one. Unlike in a movie theater, where people leave pockets of single seats rather than sit next to someone they don't know, I've noticed that at the gym, people choose to work out next to another person.

The first time someone stepped up to the treadmill next to me in an otherwise empty row of machines, I was relieved. I had assumed he would want his space or to work out next to someone more polished.

I've thought about the social aspects of fitness training often since starting on this journey. I had intended to write about this when I read about the value of peer pressure in a *New York Times* Opinionator blog entry by Helen Coster, "Peer Pressure Can Be a Lifesaver," on May 14, 2014. The author reported that in Kenya, where dirty water contributes to disease and death, a U.S.-based organization not only developed a convenient chlorine dispenser that made it simple to treat a container of water, they installed the devices where neighbors could see each other using them.

In the end, the combination of the easy-to-use, free device, and peer pressure to make use of it changed people's behavior.

"If you accept the basic framework that we make decisions to maximize our happiness, there are two parts that incorporate other people," said Yale economics professor Dean Karlan. "One part is that our happiness isn't just a function of what we eat, drink, and consume: it's also our image to others, and our reputation. The second way that people influence decisions is through their information networks. I get information from friends, and that information will affect the decisions I make. [Many public health] interventions are using those levers: They're using peers to send information."

Like a lot of social theories, this one does not seem particularly like rocket science. I mention it because I am surprised to find a neighborly atmosphere to be part of the fitness culture. Every time someone shares a tip, corrects my posture, or mentions how much they love a particular item of workout gear, I am always surprised. My own stereotype of the athletic world is framed by competitiveness, not collegiality. There's still the competitive aspect—competitiveness within yourself, and yes, with the person whose mojo you depend on running next to you—but it's friendlier than I thought it would be. Who knew?!

***

I used the Woodway treadmill at the gym on both Saturday and Sunday to focus on running and on pushing myself to run as long as possible at 5.1 MPH. I know the Woodway is the safest machine to run on, and Adorable is like a Woodway groupie, but I don't prefer it because the machines are located on the top floor of the building and fairly isolated. This relates to my comments above— you're alone when you run on the Woodway, and I find the isolation adds another level of difficulty to my workout. I am aware that listening to yourself as you run in isolation is an ultimate goal, but I am a long ways away from that one.

***

On Sunday, I drove to New Jersey to pick Adin up from college. I was loading one of his suitcases into the back of the CRV when the Honda key fell out of my shorts pocket and into the grate on the side of the road outside his dorm. I told this story to my sister Ilene at her house Sunday night during her birthday barbecue, and she got so much enjoyment picturing my face at the precise moment the key landed under the grate.

I hardly knew what to do, but despite the fact that this was not a real emergency, I dialed 911 and explained my predicament. Within a few minutes, one of New Jersey's finest drove up and pulled out a tool he uses to fish keys out of grates, because he says it happens all the time.

"I'm sorry I don't have a valet key in the glove compartment," I told him.

"Never keep a key in the glove," he reassured me. "I don't."

On the first try he retrieved the key and then let me give him a hug. It's not an overstatement to say that hug was the highlight of my day. I'm not so different from any Brownie or Girl Scout who had her first crush on a police officer in full uniform as he led the Memorial Day Parade on a motorcycle in Small Town America.

It was a nice hug.

***

One of the major perks of taking this fitness journey has been creating the time and space to listen to music. For those of us who work nine to five and hear the news or talk shows in our cars, or on the subway or bus to and from the office, there's not a lot of leisure time for listening in the way we did in high school or college, either alone in our rooms or in our friends' rooms. Last week, the gym's fitness blog featured an article on the importance of music when it comes to working out. I was talking to Adin about this and told him I thought the article was interesting but found one of the quotes bullshitty and a bit much:

"Music has a way of improving muscle coordination and aiding the muscles so they use less energy and become more effective physiologically."

"Why is that bullshit?" Adin surprised me. "Music has a beat like a heartbeat, and in that way, it very much connects and syncs with our own physical processes."

Okay then.

***

🎵 PLAYLIST HIGHLIGHTS

I looked at a few of the playlists on Beats Music, and some of this crosses with those (e.g. Tegan and Sara), but I've still got my own preferences.

Burning Down the House – Talking Heads

Boom Clap – Charli XCX

E.T. – Katy Perry (featuring Kanye West)

Empire State of Mind – Jay Z

Yeah! – Usher

OMG – Usher

Scream and Shout – DJ D.M.X.

Come on to Me – Major Lazer

Gucci – Kreayshawn

Silver Screen – Felix da Housecat

Love the Way You Lie – Eminem

After Party – Keith "Sweaty" Milgaten and Keith Stanfield

Freestyle – Bassnectar

We Run the Night – Havana Brown (I have to listen to this every time.)

Right Round – Flo Rida (This one too—you can just assume I'm listening to this genius nearly every day.)

Hey Ya! – OutKast

212 – Azealia Banks

Talk Dirty – Jason Derulo

Liquid Lunch – Caro Emerald

You Just Don't Love Me – David Morales and Tamra Keenan

It's Raining Men – The Weather Girls (Always cracks me up, and sometimes I do sing along.)

Where Does the Good Go – Tegan and Sara

Tainted Love – Soft Cell

Woods – Bon Iver

Flightless Bird – Iron and Wine

Tell It Like It Is – Aaron Neville

Day 72, June 9, 2014

> *"Ole Ole Ole Ola"*
> —Pitbull, "We Are One (Ole Ola)"

Watching the Baltimore Orioles take down the Oakland Athletics Saturday night, it was hard to picture what would happen the next day when the A's put away the O's. Even

Manny Machado's temper tantrum seemed surreal. My baseball enthusiast colleague Adam Center reminded me that every baseball team wins 60 and loses 60. The idea eludes me, but since I'm focusing on my own journey right now, I'm figuring I'm finally on the winning side of halfway.

I'm down two pounds from two weeks ago, which is still far from where I want to be, but I can check off shopping in my closet as one of my earliest little goals. Every morning I'm finding something that fits—and not a moment too soon. Adorable is my spring clothing budget, and at this point probably fall and winter, too.

It took me a few days to refocus after the Belkin family reunion. Staying away from processed sugar and sticking to no sugar within three hours of bedtime made the difference. Tightness in my chest and wheezing for most of last week kept me from running on the treadmill, but I'm working my way back up gradually to two miles at 5.1 MPH. Adorable is in Brazil for the World Cup for two weeks, so I may use the opportunity to try to run on the Capital Crescent Trail. At the suggestion of Mia's boyfriend, Julian Muller, I downloaded the MapMyRun app on my iPhone, but I'm still figuring out how to work it with my phone tucked away in a pocket or wrapped around my arm.

Tomorrow is my first session with a substitute trainer. I met Daniel Le over the weekend, and he seems perfectly nice. No one consulted me, but this is not exactly great timing for One Love One Life One World in terms of *my* training. Just when I've gotten slightly acclimated to the idea of an attractive young male fixating on every part of my body for 60 minutes, I need to think about *another* attractive young male fixating on every part of my body for 60 minutes.

I know the training culture has been around for decades and everybody seems to be onboard, but I'm slow to come around. It works, I'm committed to it, I'm wearing sleeveless dresses to work, and I don't think it would be any different if I were working with a female trainer. It's just weird. Perfectly Nice told me he has my program, but he may switch it up a bit, try some new things. Sigh.

***

For my workout day off on Sunday, I spent the morning with Adin at the Bethesda Central Farm Market and then we took a longish stroll on the Capital Crescent Trail with my mother. Later, we went to Baltimore to visit with my four-week-old nephew Bennett and his big brother, Leyton, so it was an all-around awesome day. I roasted up a pan of vegetables for lunches for the week and made a pot of ratatouille. I need to start preparing myself mentally for a series of road trips coming up, including the drive to Vassar for my reunion. I've got to come up with a strategy to keep making progress. That's on my to-do list later this week.

***

Most mornings I'm doing three miles on the recumbent bike, up to two miles running on the treadmill, six minutes on the arm bike, and floor work (leg lifts and planks). I'm seeing the difference, especially in my knees, which are more stable, and in my arms, which are no longer a scary sight.

🎵 PLAYLIST HIGHLIGHTS

We Are One (Ole Ola) – Pitbull (Of course I'm listening to the official FIFA 2014 World Cup song—I love it, so fun, and often put this on repeat on the treadmill.)

Sing – Ed Sheeran

A Sky Full of Stars – Cold Play

Latch – Disclosure

Human – Christina Perri

Come With Me Now – Kongos (I Shazamed this during the Orioles game Saturday night.)

Wild Wild Love – Pitbull

Love Never Felt So Good – Michael Jackson and Justin Timberlake (It's nice to hear Michael's voice in this.)

Best Day of My Life – American Authors

We Run the Night – Havana Brown

The Boxer – Mumford and Sons

I Will Wait – Mumford and Sons

m.A.A.d city – Kendrick Lamar

All I Do Is Win – DJ Khaled

Yeah! – Usher

OMG – Usher

Day 81, June 18, 2014

"Feels like home."

—Dolly Parton, Linda Ronstadt &
Emmy Lou Harris, "Feels Like Home"

Attending my Vassar reunion last weekend was kind of like how I feel about the Prius. I like the idea of a Prius, and I don't have a problem with Prius owners, I just don't like driving behind one.

Ripped looked gorgeous, healthy, and happy, as did a few others, especially the women. And overall most of my classmates looked nearly as good as the campus, which according to at least two people looked "so fucking good," which gives you an idea of where some of us are at.

I loved being back at Vassar, but it reminded me how young I was then and how much time has passed. I'm trying not to dwell on this, and I know it's not about looking good. The truth is, it was the time of my life and a great place to be young and open-minded, and I doubt I thought about my physical well-being for more than five minutes in four years. Overthinking is the stuff of reunions, so I expect I'm in good company.

I don't like to complain about food when someone else prepares it for me, but I was surprised and dismayed at how old school the dining hall food was, especially when I know colleges everywhere are fairly enlightened about the mind / body connection to developing brains. After meeting Donna

Balmuth, my classmate Keith Loris's wife, for an hour-long walk to Sunset Lake and the Walker Field House at six in the morning, I could not find anything reasonably healthy to eat for breakfast in the dining hall on Saturday except for half a grapefruit. It was like time had stood still; I could have been at Denny's.

Being in college is like living in a protective bubble, but I still think it's worth taking a peek outside to see what's out there. I asked if they had any hard-boiled eggs, and the kitchen worker seemed genuinely sorry that the answer was no. By Sunday, though, there was a basket of hard-boiled eggs, so that with the grapefruit and a piece of whole wheat toast worked fine.

The air had become chilly overnight, so after Donna and I finished our walk on Sunday morning, this time trying to somehow find an opening in the fence surrounding Prentiss Field, which wasn't going to happen, I decided to try to take a shot at running. I opened the MapMyRun app, and before taking off, I noticed I could link my music to my run. I got a kick out of exploring the campus this way as I looped around the science and theater buildings, because I can say with 100 percent certainty, even if I don't remember everything that went on during my four years at Vassar, I know I never broke a sweat running around outside. I made it back to Jewett and looked to see how much I had run. Oops, I had neglected to click "resume my run" after selecting my music, so the only way to find out was to do the route a second time. I couldn't figure out how to shuffle an individual playlist, so I was shuffling among all of the songs on my phone, including the cantor reciting Adin's bar mitzvah portion.

When I checked in again and "Feels Like Home" was playing, I had run .97 miles. How crazy is that? At the very first opportunity, my plan is to run from my house down Connecticut Ave to Chevy Chase Circle (1.5 miles) and then run or walk back. I'm not sure when I'll get to this since I've got another big road trip coming up to Minneapolis, where I've booked hotels along the way with good fitness centers, but it's on my mind.

***

About halfway into this journey, my colleague Ambassador Susan Jacobs, who takes staying fit to a whole other level as she travels the globe, told me she works out so she can eat. She brings her fitness regimen with her wherever she is every day. On one trip to Rome where we flew in separately—she from at least a week in Africa and me in from an overnight flight from Washington—I got a call from her three minutes after she checked in to our hotel.

"Let's take a walk."

My head was already on the pillow.

Susan and I recently traveled to Turkey with Beth Cooper, another colleague, who just broke her ankle. She came into work wearing a boot, and the first thing she told us was how stressed she was about not being able to work out. I'm super focused on results and avoiding injury, and I'm still eating to work out versus working out to eat, but I keep reminding myself how happy I am to be a member of this club. And how much I need this: to get better sleep, to fit into better clothes, to have a better day at work.

Just better.

***

I was called in for randomized drug testing last week for the first time since joining the State Department in 2005. Once you get the call, you have two hours to report for the test.

"Make sure you drink something before you come in, because we'll need to get a urine specimen," I heard the person say as I rolled my eyes on the other end of the phone.

Duh.

I told my team I'd be back in about 30 minutes and headed to the Department of the Interior building a few blocks from my office in Foggy Bottom. I checked in and followed the instructions, but when I went into the bathroom to provide the specimen, I could not fill the cup to the black line. I hadn't expected such a big cup.

Now I'd have to stay within the secure part of the building and come up with a sample within three hours. There were two other petite women in the same situation, and another was waiting to take her test who told us this had also happened to her the last time. She said it had taken her the full three hours, and now she was under considerable stress. In the meantime, big people were coming in and out so fast we started to feel self-conscious.

I drink so much water during the day that I'm in the bathroom constantly. Seriously.

And I had to concentrate on de-stressing so as not to undo my morning workout by producing cortisol and releasing sugar and fat into my bloodstream.

I started filling up little cups of water and drinking as quickly as I could, but then one of the drug-testing staff told me to stop. "Once they test the sample, if it's diluted it'll be invalid."

He told us to speed walk up and down the hallways and to do jumping jacks. He said one of the personal trainers would be by shortly with a jump rope. I didn't want to stick around to find out if he wasn't joking.

I used my lifeline and texted Lord Baltimore.

"Diet Coke."

A staff member graciously agreed to escort me to a vending machine.

The whole thing took two hours, but the Diet Coke worked, and I shared it with the others. I still can't fathom why they need so much, but the moment I hit the black line, I removed all of this from my brain, and until now it's been like it never existed.

***

My overnight shift in the Department's Operations Center was canceled late on Monday, so I immediately made a

6 p.m. appointment at Blue Zen in Bethesda for a manicure/ pedicure. I had already downloaded Watch ESPN on my iPhone, so as I sat in the pedi-chair and hit the power button on the massage feature, I caught that first goal in the U.S.A. v. Ghana World Cup game. I especially appreciated the replay, because there's only one thing worse than watching the World Cup on television, and that's watching it on a three-inch screen. I'm not a soccer fan, and I don't know much about the game, but it's hard not to get swept away by it all.

After my appointment, I watched the game in my kitchen before leaving for a late dinner to celebrate my nephew Harry Slonim's high school graduation just in time to see Ghana score. Then I rushed to my car, but by the time I found the ESPN station, I had missed the U.S.A. goal at 86 minutes in. Still, so exciting and what a thrill!

***

I haven't been able to be structured with my workouts since I've been traveling. I've been back at the gym for early morning cardio this week and doing my favorite regimen, but in an abbreviated form, since I'm sleeping in, too: two miles on the recumbent bike, one mile running on the treadmill, five minutes on the arm bike, and core work on the floor. I have a training session tomorrow morning, which I hope will jumpstart my workouts on the road this weekend.

🎵 PLAYLIST HIGHLIGHTS

I'm shuffling between my up-to-date favorites and oldies, including Pink Floyd and Rod Stewart, which the high-energy Pilates instructor played during the class I took at Vassar on Saturday and the DJ in Matthew's Mug played Friday night.

Feels Like Home – Dolly Parton, Linda Ronstadt, and Emmy Lou Harris

Sweet Dreams – Eurythmics

Maggie May – Rod Stewart

Money – Pink Floyd

Family Affair – Mary J. Blige

Sunday Morning – Maroon 5

We Are One (Ole Ola) – Pitbull

Latch – Disclosure

Come With Me Now – Kongos

I Am the Best – 2NE1

Sabali – Amadou and Mariam

Coastin' – Zion I & K. Flay

Down with the Trumpets – Rizzle Kicks

The Other Side – Jason Derulo

Gucci Gucci – Kreayshawn

Silver Screen – Felix da Housecat

We Run the Night – Havana Brown

Empire State of Mind – Alicia Keys

Rhythm of Love – Plain White Ts

Day 90, June 27, 2014

> *"This boat will stay afloat."*
> —Travie McCoy, "Rough Water"

I never intended for my doctor's office to be the place where I weigh in every few weeks, but there I was back again on Wednesday with what presented like sciatica. The good news is that at least for now, my doctor ruled out any lower back or spinal / disc issues, and I've lost two more pounds.

The bad news is he prescribed physical therapy, and my really smart physical therapist, Dr. Katie Taraban Mahoney at Elite Physical Therapy and Wellness in upper Georgetown, whom I'm now seeing two times a week, says I'm presenting more like a hamstring strain and has taken me off the treadmill. Running has been a key factor in my weight loss, so I'm bummed. Even Ripped agreed last night on the margins of our book group discussion of the fiftieth anniversary of *The Feminine Mystique* that she thinks running has made all the difference in her own weight loss.

Really Smart gave me a ton of stretching and rehab exercises to do at home and at the gym, and she did both dry needling and "stim," or electrical stimulation.

The idea behind dry needling, which uses needles without injecting any kind of medication, is to release trigger points in the muscle that may be knotted. I had seen Wonderful on Tuesday night for deep tissue massage, which is basically the same thing, except needles can get even deeper into the muscle to relieve any tension. I felt a thousand times better after seeing Wonderful, so you can imagine how uncomfortable I was if I felt that much better after the needles and stim. Seriously, it's not like I'm an athlete, so I understand why major league baseball players are often out on the disabled list for hamstring strain. It's painful.

I'm not sure what stim does, but it felt like the machine was sending electrical currents through my leg over a heated blanket. At times the stimulation was too much, but the warmth felt good. The needles hurt at first, rather like a twinge in the muscle, but after a few seconds I was fine.

Let me pause for a moment to reflect on how shockingly relaxed I've become with having multiple people digging for knots and tension in my buttocks and thighs. I've clearly lost all sense of inhibition, which I'm thinking is a good thing.

As the day wore on yesterday, I was feeling increasingly better, but when I woke up this morning, the pain—starting in my glute and running down my thigh—was as bad as ever. Really Smart said soreness after needles is normal, so I did some gentle stretching at home and took some Tylenol, and since I had already decided today was going to be my workout day off, tried hard to focus on developing a strategy to (1) get results and (2) get endorphins.

I can swim.

It's as if all the experts I'm working with—Adorable, my knee doctor, my internist, Wonderful, and Really Smart are conspiring to throw me into the pool, which is my least favorite place to be.

"You can swim."

I don't even put water on my face. It's like Neutrogena face wipes were invented for me, and swimming laps, even in the pleasing salt water pool at the gym, is a visceral reminder of my coming of age in Long Island, where I threw up after nearly every swim team practice.

I should be grateful I know *how* to swim, but I do not want to swim. I swam Wednesday morning and powered through 45 minutes doing 50 meters in 50 seconds, and I got a great endorphin rush that lasted for several hours. But I also spent most of the day with goggle marks around my eyes and frizzy hair.

And thinking out loud here, *how's this supposed to work exactly?*

I still need to do 20 minutes on the recumbent bike in order to strengthen the muscles around my knees, and following Really Smart's guidance, I absolutely have to do the arm bike for at least six minutes in order to make progress on destroying the not-so-lovely Hello Betty thriving under my upper arms; and as I've got a beach vacation coming up way before I'd scheduled to be beach-body ready, I need to be on the mat working my core.

So, do I get in the pool first, and then rinse off in the shower and head up to the training area and then back down to the showers? Or do I use the bikes, do the floor work, and then get in the pool? What about stretching? I've learned it's better to warm the muscles before working out and stretch them after. So, when is after? After what?

Between practically daily training and working out at the gym, visits to the doctor, and now physical therapy, the registered dietician, biweekly massage therapy, and picking up supplies during business hours at R and J Running and City Sports, and showing up for work to support all of this, I'm standing by my earlier statement that if I wasn't getting a rush and having some fun, I'd have every reason to stop right now.

♬ PLAYLIST HIGHLIGHTS

Here's what I'm listening to in the pool—mostly some of my favorite hip-hop oldies.

Latch – Disclosure

Come With Me Now – Kongos

We Are One (Ole Ola) – Pitbull (I'm still loving this.)

Pump It – Black Eyed Peas

Lean Back – Terror Squad

Rough Water – Travie McCoy

Mockingbird – Eminem

Let's Get It Started – Black Eyes Peas

Where'd You Go – Fort Minor

Wouldn't Have It Any Other Way – The Streets

Switch – Will Smith

Where Is the Love – Black Eyed Peas

We Be Burnin' – Sean Paul

Lose Yourself – Eminem

Temperature – Sean Paul

The Boogie That Be – Black Eyed Peas

Club Can't Handle Me – Flo Rida

Hard Knock Life – Jay Z

Sexy and I Know It – LMFAO

Envy – 116 Man Up

No Church in the Wild – Kanye and Jay Z

Sunshine – Mos Def

Crazy Kids – Kesha

The Way I Are – Timbaland

Hey Ya! – Outkast

Coastin' – Zion I and K. Flay

Down with the Trumpets – Rizzle Kicks

Right Round – Flo Rida

Timber – Pitbull

CHAPTER 3 – REUEL

When I met Carolee, I had only been training clients for three months. My first goal was to understand where she was coming from.

I had reached out to her a few times after another trainer had tried to get her to come in for an assessment.

We emailed back and forth, and as I was about to give up, she said she'd come in to meet me.

My first impression of Carolee was, *where are her shoes?*

She said she'd forgotten them, but when I told her that wouldn't be a problem, that we'd be able to complete most of the assessments, she did not seem upset.

My second impression of Carolee?

She's easygoing.

And then I wondered, *when was the last time she had a consistent exercise regimen?*

We talked about her goals, and she let me know she had tried a few sessions with another trainer at another gym but felt that was a bust because the trainer continued to push exercises Carolee felt weren't right for her. She told me she had tried an open line of communication with that trainer but had ultimately given up, even though she had paid for a package and was throwing away sessions.

Pretty quickly I realized that in order to help her get to where she wanted to go, I would have to make sure she felt comfortable.

This is something I try to do with everyone. I wanted Carolee to trust me. In order for her to make gains, I needed her to understand exactly what we were doing and why. We needed to have a rapport. I knew if I didn't explain the exercises to her, I wasn't going to get her buy-in.

Carolee told me her goal was to lose weight. She mentioned an important black-tie event coming up, and she had a particular dress she wanted to wear. When she told me the event was only a few weeks away, I said that in that time frame we could get started, but her goal wasn't going to happen.

I wanted to help her achieve her goal, but at same time I didn't want her to think it was going to happen immediately. I was very upfront because I wanted her to take me seriously.

We needed to be on the same page.

At our initial session after the assessment, Carolee told me that she did not want to bulk up and that she was reluctant to work with weights. I explained to her the role that weights play in building muscle, and how building muscle can speed up the body's ability to burn calories.

Carolee wasn't buying it, and even though I didn't agree with her, I was still learning myself and knew there are many ways of getting around certain pieces of equipment in order to achieve the same goal.

I thought this might be an interesting and challenging learning experience. I wanted to help her progress but at the same time keep her engaged and interested so she wouldn't stop working with me.

In order to make Carolee feel comfortable, I developed a program for her using bands and tubing. I knew it would take a few months to see results, and I had never worked with bands or tubes before, but I felt confident.

In order to do complete sessions without weights or machines, I had to sit down and write out my programs for her. I spent more time developing her programs than I was used to because I was more comfortable training with weights and machines. Most of the time machines are especially appropriate for beginners because they're not complicated and can only go in one direction.

One particular arm exercise we did with tubing was so complicated that I remember Carolee staring at me as I wrapped tubing around anything I could find nearby.

We used bands and tubing for a few months. I was trying to get Carolee to execute correct form and technique, while she was getting used to the feeling of fatiguing and having her muscles burn. I sensed her frustration, but I chose not to focus on it.

My job was to get her where she wanted, and I was going to try to make her extremely comfortable with the idea of exercising. I agreed not to use weights, but I wasn't going to pamper her. She needed to get comfortable with that idea too.

When we first started working together, her core was weak, and I could tell she was pushing too hard. Often, I had to stop her, because I knew if I didn't and she became overwhelmed, she'd never come back.

That's when we'd take a break. Later, as her workouts intensified, I thought, *Okay, we're getting somewhere. We're building a solid base.*

For beginners like Carolee, performing and executing exercises correctly can take a lot of energy and focus. If you're not used to this, it can feel a lot worse than it actually is.

I didn't think Carolee was going to pass out or collapse, but I could tell she was contemplating whether she wanted to continue.

Carolee's perspective on weight loss was not uncommon. The number one issue why people go to the gym is because of their weight.

It's easy to lose track of how much exercise you're doing or how many calories you're consuming because of everything else going on in your life. But to do the opposite and work

hard to change your eating habits and exercise regularly—
then it's a 180-degree turnaround as you see results.

As I got to know Carolee, I realized this was going to be
good and we were going to have some fun with this. For
anything physical, you need to have mental strength to
work toward what you're doing, and we talked a lot about
this. All of us have certain senses that tell us to stop, and
for people who haven't worked out intensively, it's hard to
know where that line is.

At the beginning, I was dead serious when I told Carolee
she needed to train four days a week. I told her she needed
to do a lot on her own and call me or text me with any
questions or concerns. I also told her she needed to walk
two miles every day.

I knew I could help her, but at same time she would have to
do a lot on her own.

CHAPTER 4 –
IF I LOOK LIKE A
DIFFERENT PERSON,
IT'S BECAUSE I AM

Day 98, July 5, 2014

> *"I can't say what life will show me,*
> *but I know what I've seen."*
> —Jimmy Cliff, "Sitting in Limbo"

I'm under an umbrella with my toes in the sand in Ocho Rios, in Saint Ann's Parish, Jamaica. I've been here before, but every time I return I'm moved by the natural beauty of the place and the people. I know it's important to visit new places, but this is where I want to be.

Part of it is the music, of course. Calypso, reggae, rasta—as intoxicating as the fresh mint infusing my single mojito of the day. We got a dose of Jamaican politics from our driver on the way from Montego Bay to Ocho Rios while passing through pockets of abject poverty and herds of goats.

Without any hesitation or self-consciousness, the driver refers to Jamaica as "third world." The temperature at this time of year is nearly ninety degrees, and it doesn't cool down much in the evenings. We're comfortable on the beach and under ceiling fans during meals served in rooms open to the sea, but the air conditioner runs cool all night in our room while we sleep. Most of the homes we passed on our drive did not have screens or glass on the windows, so it's safe to say there are no air conditioners.

Yet from the moment you arrive in Montego Bay, which, like Negril and Ocho Rios, thrives on tourism, you are greeted by people who despite living in a developing country give off an unmistakable happiness vibe. I know that's a big generalization, and tourism is a smallish part of a larger economy focused on the hard work of coffee, sugar, and almond farms, but with all of that understood, it is impossible to be unmoved by the Jamaican smile.

"Ya mon."

"Soon come."

On the plane I was reading the latest issue of *More* magazine—the one with Lisa Kudrow on the cover—where I came across a piece on neuropsychologist Rick Hanson's new book, *Hardwiring Happiness: The New Brain Science of Contentment, Calm, and Confidence.*

Hanson's thesis is that the human brain has a natural negativity bias. He says from the time of our evolution in the Stone Age we've trained ourselves to let good experiences bounce off the brain while bad ones go right in.

He says we can train ourselves to alter the bias so we can be happier. For example, we can register a simple good experience, such as by feeling relaxed as we exhale or by looking at a beautiful tree. Or we can think about someone in our life who cares about us. So that's the first step— activating a positive mental state.

It only counts if you look at the beautiful tree and consciously register it as a positive experience. The next step is to dwell on the positive experience by staying completely aware of it for about twelve seconds. Hanson says to try to enrich the experience by accessing different senses. For example, if you're outside your house standing by the beautiful tree, inhale the scent of the soil and feel a slight breeze cross your face. His point is that by prolonging and enriching the positive memory, you'll get as many neurons as possible to start firing so they can wire together.

Once you train yourself to consciously absorb the positive experience or to tell yourself you are absorbing the positive experience, the payoff is you'll begin to create new neural connections that transform passing mental states, such as feeling cheerful, into lasting neural traits, i.e., being a cheerful person.

Maybe this is what happens subconsciously to people who live amid incredible natural beauty. I suspected this when I lived in the San Francisco Bay Area, and I'm wondering if this is what is happening in Jamaica.

At the end of a long travel day yesterday, we changed into our bathing suits after dinner and took a late-night swim in the pool. Nearby, the old-timers in the calypso band played Bob Marley's intensely poignant and personal "Redemption Song," which some say is the unofficial Jamaican national anthem.

"Emancipate yourselves from mental slavery/None but ourselves can free our minds."

What I know about the song is that Marley wrote it when he was beginning to face his own mortality after he was diagnosed with cancer. But when I listened to it last night, I was thinking about Hanson's ideas of training our brains to register the good instead of the bad.

This is my work this week on a beautiful beach in Jamaica.

***

After two and a half weeks and five two-hour sessions of physical therapy, including five dry needling treatments, my strained hamstring is on the mend. Adorable and Really Smart are talking with each other and coordinating to ensure its progress. At first my reaction to this was, *There's only one thing worse than a single person focused on your body, and that's two people focused and talking to each other about your body.*

But after reading about Hanson's theories, I'm filled with an overall sense of happiness as I contemplate two professionals who care about me, talking to each other about me on my behalf. They are both really smart and both completely adorable, but they are so much more than smart and adorable.

***

This morning after my workout day off yesterday, I waded in the turquoise blue water on my way to the fitness center. I did 30 minutes on the recumbent bike, and with Really Smart's okay and Adorable's guidance, 30 minutes on the elliptical, which I loved. Really Smart told me I could then move into a gentle jog on the treadmill if I felt okay. Of course, you know I did, and then after one mile at 4.5 MPH on the treadmill I felt more than okay. I felt great.

And I remembered to register the feeling.

Day 100, July 7, 2014

> *"Let's ride still stayn' low-key."*
> —Ground Up, "Let's Ride"

I'm thinking about what I'm eating all the time. Since injuring my hamstring, I'm consciously bringing in more lean protein and fewer carbs. This takes willpower because like everyone else I naturally gravitate toward carbs. Here in Jamaica, where seafood is available at every meal, I'm having an easier time choosing protein.

Breakfast this morning after our workout included ackee— the national fruit of Jamaica—and lobster served with a boiled white yam, also native to Jamaica, a boiled banana, and a Johnny cake—a dense piece of fried dough that tastes more like a beignet than you would think by working hard to slice through it. I skipped the Johnny cake, because as with beignets, I figure I've already had a lifetime's share of donuts of any kind.

What to do with all that lobster? Lord Baltimore smiled just thinking about the chef's daily dilemma.

Yesterday I had poached eggs with sliced tomatoes and steamed callaloo, some kind of kale-like leafy vegetable, served on top of an English muffin—a modified Eggs Florentine. The stack didn't need the English muffin, so I slid it off my plate. Instead, I added mango and papaya quarters. After living in California where mangoes and papayas were available year-round, I had developed a taste for tropical fruits; I'm able to get good papayas in Washington, but finding great mangoes is not easy. Here in Jamaica, where canopy nets cover the property to catch falling mangoes, I don't think I could choose anything better to put on my plate than a naturally ripened mango.

Ackee is usually served with "salt fish"—maybe like a cod— but this dish is reserved for special occasions and Sundays. We had this yesterday, and although the ackee and lobster tasted great this morning, the salt fish gave the fruit a little more balance. I asked our waitress if I could order the ackee on its own, and she said it doesn't have a good flavor without the fish. To me, although the texture of the ackee is creamy, I think it resembles the part of the Maryland blue crab we typically discard. Delicious, but it takes some getting used to, aesthetically speaking.

So much of the food here is perfectly spiced. Twice I've had escoveitch, which is hot peppery seasoned red snapper, and it's hard to consider you'd ever get tired of eating anything jerked, especially jerked shrimp. But as a result, I'm not finding wines that work with these spices.

Ironically, the best and only food pairing class I've ever taken was given by a French chef right here in Ocho Rios a few years ago. One takeaway is to pair sweeter wines with spicier foods, such as Thai or other Asian foods, for example, with a Gewürztraminer or a Riesling. This works back home in Washington at a Thai place that serves maybe a dry Gewürztraminer from California, but here in Jamaica after I've been off refined sugar for weeks now, even the pink Zinfandel seems too sugary. After trying some Italian whites, I'm sticking with sparkling wine with a touch of freshly squeezed mango juice. Lord Baltimore is drinking vodka with freshly squeezed tropical juices with dinner instead of wine, so I think he's having the same natural inclinations. There's always Red Stripe, which to me works better with jerked pork than with grilled lobster or jerked shrimp.

***

Just before we left Washington, my sister Phyllis Belkin sent me a link to Nina Manolson's Nourished Woman Nation. I've only had a chance to get slightly acquainted with the blog, but I'm thinking the group conference calls and recipes might be valuable.

My sense is that Manolson, a self-described food psychologist, taps into the whole discussion of metabolism as we age, and she also points us in better directions using foods we may not have paid any attention to even a few years ago. (My sister is serving her family pudding made from chia seeds that she says does a good job looking and tasting like traditional tapioca, for example.)

***

Although I'm obviously listening to island music all week, I did get the chance to hear "Let's Ride" by Philadelphia rap artist Ground Up. Everything people are saying about this song is true—it's great.

Day 113, July 20, 2014

> *"The zone, own, yes I'm in the zone."*
> —Nicki Minaj, "Starships"

What bothers me about Tom Junod's article in *Esquire* in praise of older women is not his sexualization of women. I'm okay with being sexualized as long as I'm the one doing the sexualizing. It's Junod's tired objectification of women that defines us in the context of our ability to arouse men. This is not a subtle point, as I am not talking about the sexual revolution, which persisted in placing women in the context of stimulating men. It's #yesallwomen all over again.

"Let's face it," Junod writes, "there used to be something tragic about even the most beautiful forty-two-year-old woman. With half her life still ahead of her, she was deemed to be at the end of something—namely, everything society valued in her, other than her success as a mother. If she remained sexual, she was either predatory or desperate; if she remained beautiful, what gave her beauty force was the fact of its fading. And if she remained alone...well, then God help her."

Junod goes on to say that with a lot of yoga and Pilates, women in their forties are looking hotter than ever.

"The best thing that forty-two-year-old American men have going for them is forty-two-year-old American women."

So, what is Junod talking about here? Because he's not talking about the sexually healthy men and women I know. It's a widely held rumor that men think about sex every seven seconds, which adds up to 514 times per hour or about 7,200 times a day while they're awake, and I don't even want to think about how this number fits into a guy's sleep cycle.

Contemplating this, Tom Stafford writing for the BBC, asks how it's possible for anyone to count the number of a person's thoughts, let alone whether we are able to count our own over the course of a day. He looked at a study at Ohio State that gave clickers to college students and asked them to record each time they thought about sex, food, or sleep. The results showed that on average, the males in the study had 19 thoughts a day about sex versus the females, who had 10. But the males also had a larger number of thoughts about food and sleep than women, so maybe, the researchers surmised, males have more indulgent thoughts each day than females overall.

Over the course of the day I think about sex, but I also think about shoes and exfoliating. I'm sure I don't spend any time thinking about whether my sex appeal is arousing men.

Seriously, do men think they are arousing women during the course of a work day or on the street or the Metro?

Feminism has always been about equality—equal opportunity as well as equal choice—and while women have achieved a certain amount of equality, including finally health equality, there are apparently scores of individuals such as Junod who are confused by women who exude sexual health. I don't think any of us knows anything about the sexual health of the forty-two-year-old celebrities Junod focuses on—Sofia Vergara and Cameron Diaz, for example—by studying their screen personalities, but the "together" women I know have the total package of health and well-being. I'm fine with "look hot, stay cool" or "sexy abs fast" cover stories in recent issues of *Women's Running*, because looking hot while staying cool and having six-pack abs are part of my goals to be physically, mentally, and sexually healthy. (Yes, I know how crazy it is that I subscribe to *Women's Running*. Even crazier that I subscribe to *Runner's World*, too.)

If we exude confidence and sex appeal, it's because we have a healthy approach to our own sexuality that at its core is about consensuality.

This is why college campuses are establishing zero tolerance policies for rape when sex is not consensual. Even if it's a woman's (poor) choice to drink too much, if the sex is not consensual, it's rape. When I was in my twenties, we talked about rape being an act of violence, not sex. Today I think it's both an act of power and an act of unhealthy sex. One of the characters investigating the gang rape of a fellow soldier serving in Iraq in the play *One Night* by playwright Charles Fuller, which I saw today at the Contemporary American Theater Festival in Shepherdstown, tells the victim he believes her, but he's never been in favor of women serving in combat side by side with men

"If you hadn't been there, this wouldn't have happened."

Like the army colonel, Junod persists in asserting that women are responsible for men's arousal and one may extrapolate any nonconsensual acts that follow. I am so not into men remotely like Junod, and am completely exhausted by the idea that women are somehow responsible for the cat calls on the street when they're out jogging in Under Armour compressionwear. From looking at Junod's photo, I hope he has someone in his life who loves him truly, madly, deeply, because unless I'm missing something, he has no appeal whatsoever.

Charles Clymer, who blogs for the *Huffington Post,* writes that although "linguistically, 'woman' is not another word for sex...culturally, the two couldn't be more intertwined." He points out that as a man his worldview is free of sexual restraint:

> *My successes are my own, not because*
> *I supposedly slept with someone.*
>
> *My medical issues aren't tied to their*
> *sexual importance.*
>
> *The credibility of my opinion isn't based on*
> *the sexual identity of those listening.*
>
> *My concerns are supposedly based on logical*
> *reasoning, not hormone-induced emotion.*
>
> *The world is my sex-assumption-free oyster,*
> *unless I choose otherwise.*

—Charles Clymer

As the 16-week mark approaches on August 1 of my get-fit journey, Adorable continues to remind me that results are about how I feel and not about the numbers on the scale or even how I look (although that's stretching it). I'm no longer obsessed with the scale, even if I am still a teeny bit focused on it, and I so want six-pack abs. But what I finally get is that this journey, which goes way beyond 16 weeks, is absolutely about how I feel because it's about my health, my mental and physical well-being, and my sexual health.

"I've learned that people will forget what you said, people will forget what you did, but people will never forget how you made them feel." The late Maya Angelou had it right. How I feel matters, both to me and how I relate to others. How I feel about myself is very much intertwined with how much of a positive connection I am able to make with friends, colleagues, and strangers.

***

The last time I finished a highly emotional book in an overly public place, I was gasping for air as I sobbed my way through *A Thousand Splendid Suns* on a crowded Vamoose bus from Bethesda to New York. Not a pretty sight, but I couldn't help myself.

Last Saturday, after returning from a relaxing beach vacation in Jamaica, I wept on the recumbent bike at Equinox as I finished *Me Before You,* the incredibly funny but moving story of a British woman and her relationship as a caregiver to a quadriplegic man. I can't do this very often, because I find myself slumping further and further into the seat, so that by the time I'm practically on the floor, I've slowed to something just short of a pause. My sister Ilene recommended this one. She said she knew it didn't sound much like a beach book but that it was well written and had more emotional depth than you would expect in a pleasure read. Take a look at it. I also read *The Interestings,* which both Mia and Adin recommended, and it was also a great read. Now I'm finishing up *Americanah,* which is as good as everyone says it is.

***

My workouts in Jamaica and since I've returned have focused on getting myself back up to speed on cardio work, including now the elliptical, which I'm totally enjoying, and running, even at a slower pace averaging 4.5–5.0 MPH. In the middle of the week, I was back to two miles on the treadmill, and I'm doing 45 minutes on the elliptical. Training sessions are extremely focused right now, cycling between upper-body, core, and lower body, and each session, for me at least, is taking the whole idea of training up a notch. I'm only now able to lift a bag of peaches after Thursday's upper-body work. I'm still seeing Really Smart for physical therapy, but my hamstring is much improved.

***

PLAYLIST HIGHLIGHTS

A mix of reggae and oldies (not sure why I'm listening to these, but hopefully I'll have gotten them through my system within a few more days).

Kingston Town – UB40

Red Red Wine – UB40

You're Beautiful – James Blunt

Sweat (Alalalalalalong) – Inner Circle (I pretend this is about working out.)

Real Jamaican – Busy Signal

Redemption Song – Bob Marley

Lepo Lepo – Santana and Wyclef

Pressure Drop – Toots and the Maytals

Sitting in Limbo – Jimmy Cliff

Electric Avenue – Eddy Grant

Drop Baby Drop – Eddy Grant

Maggie May – Rod Stewart

Money – Pink Floyd

Family Affair – Mary J. Blige

Losing My Religion – REM

Baby, I Love Your Way – Peter Frampton

I Know You Want Me – Pitbull

Starships – Nicki Minaj

Miss You – Rolling Stones

Day 118, July 25, 2014

> *"It's hard to catch the light."*
> —Colony House, "Silhouettes"

The hardest thing for me about traveling, especially going through different time zones and waiting for connections in airports, is making smart food choices when it feels like each day has at least eight meals.

It's limited what you can get through security—you can't bring your own water or yogurt, for example—and who wants to carry a lunch bag and a cool pack that you'll need to lug around for the rest of your trip?

I've been able to fill small sandwich bags with blueberries and almonds, and I found a Potbelly at Dulles that makes veggie chickpea salad, but other than that, I feel like I am a captive surrounded by foods I never eat.

I was reading the food journals of women who have lost one hundred pounds in *People*, and it struck me that all of them say they have between six and eight small meals per day as part of their daily regimen.

The meals are what you would expect—a breakfast scramble with egg whites and spinach, or veggies and salad greens with a protein for lunch, for example. It's almost impossible to eat this way when you're traveling, and on top of that, it's incredibly boring to sit still waiting to board your flight, waiting for your flight to take off, waiting for your flight to touch down, waiting for your luggage *blah blah blah*. All of this boredom and waiting works up an appetite, and before you've arrived at your destination and met your family or friends for dinner, you've already had between six and eight small meals.

And then your mind goes to the victims of the Malaysia 17 and Malaysia 370 disasters and their families, and it's hard to put into words how helpless you start to feel. Bring on the cortisol.

***

Recently, I've had to find a way to keep my focus. I'm even having trouble getting in my zone during training, and I've found myself leaving the gym feeling disappointed with myself. I know everyone has a bad week, but my bad week's lasting more than seven days.

I don't want to whine, but I've also got to deal with a hamstring strain that is better one day and worse the next. And now the IT band and my quad on the same leg are making it difficult to make progress. I'm still able to run at a comfortable pace, and the elliptical doesn't bother me, but any kind of strengthening workout that touches my left hamstring, glute, or quad is hard to push through, although critical to do.

I'm using Kinesio tape, which seems to help the soreness. The tape is also stabilizing my hamstring, so I can get through the airport fashionably in my summer wedges. Even if I feel like crap, at least I am looking good, which I'm not embarrassed to admit goes a long way.

🎵 PLAYLIST HIGHLIGHTS

One upside to sitting around in airports is taking time to discover new music. Here's some of what I'm listening to as I wait for my Chicago connection to Minneapolis.

Silhouettes – Colony House

Runaway Baby – Bruno Mars

Let's Ride – Ground Up

Weezer – Island in the Sun (I listened to their new album *Everything Will Be Alright In The End*, but I'm not crazy about it and went back to this oldie.)

Beck – Morning Phase (I found snippets of Beck's recent album Song Reader.)

Day 128, August 4, 2014

> *"To my heartbeat sound."*
> —Calvin Harris, "Summer"

It doesn't feel like a lot of time has passed, but when you write it down, 128 looks like a lot of days between Day 1 and now.

It has been sixteen weeks since I began this journey, which has included small side trips and distractions, and Adorable was right: I'm starting to see results. I feel like I could fit my body into where it was on Day 1, and my total weight loss so far (after lots of ups and downs) is exactly 10 pounds. Not a huge number, but possibly halfway to my goal weight, since I'm not 100 percent certain what that will be until I get there.

If I look like a different person, it's because I am.

While professionally I'm still working full time, and more during a crisis, I am doing very little of what I did before Day 1.

1. I'm not watching any television. I know there is great television out there, but I can't fit it in right now, so *Scandal* and *The Bachelor* will have to wait.

2. I'm not reading for pleasure. I caught up when I was in Jamaica, but by the time I walk into the house at close to nine o'clock in the evening, I am physically not able to sync my eyes with my brain.

3.   I'm using social media to keep up with current
     events. I've subscribed to the new NYT mobile
     app, where I get a morning and evening briefing
     delivered to me with what I need to know. I read
     these briefings on my iPhone during warm ups
     whether I'm at the gym for training or cardio. The
     briefings disappear if you don't access them, so you
     don't feel guilty about a big pile of unread papers
     or magazines. I also follow *Huffington Post* and
     Breaking News on Twitter with notifications coming
     straight into my phone, so if I see something I have
     to read, I can get to it while I'm warming up. I'm
     generally way behind on *This American Life*,
     The Splendid Table, and *Fresh Air* podcasts, but
     after two road trips to Minneapolis and back, I'm
     up-to-date.

4.   I'm not spending money on clothing except athletic
     wear. Lately I'm totally into sleeveless tanks and
     have found Nike's Dri-FIT racer tank to be close
     to perfect. I have a few pairs of Under Armour
     bottoms, which are half the price of Lululemons,
     but I don't wear them for training because they are
     oddly slippery. I'm working out six days a week,
     sometimes twice a day, so it's in everyone's best
     interest for me to have an abundance of gear.

5.   I am not eating for pleasure. I am strategic about
     getting the foods I need at the right time, but
     I am enjoying cooking and baking new things
     and thinking about foods in this way. I sent in a

question to the Nourished Woman Nation July coaching call about what to eat before and after workouts because I'm still experimenting with this. At first, I was annoyed with Nina Manolson's response: Practice "attuned eating." But I've become attuned to everything else related to my body, so why not what I eat? She has a point. I'm using my being-in-the-moment yoga skills to help me tune in to what I think my body needs, and then that's what I'm eating. That may mean an egg for dinner, but if that's what I've got ready to go and it's what I need, then I have an egg for dinner.

6. I am no longer self-conscious or in any way inhibited at the gym. Whether I've got pools of sweat dripping from my chin or I need to close my eyes and zone out, I'm not concerned about it.

I was reading one of the articles in my daily briefing written by a techie who had checked into the Fitness Ranch for two months. I didn't bookmark the article, so I can't find it quickly now, but I remember agreeing with one of his tips: be social. At the gym especially, I am friendly with everyone. I'm always working out next to someone, and I've allowed my body language to indicate that I am willing to acknowledge him or her. Now that I'm up on the rolling culture—which by the way, is it just me, or is it such a good idea mashing your muscles?—I enjoy unplugging and chatting it up.

So where am I now? I did my first run on the Capital Crescent Trail on Sunday (2.12 miles!) I enjoyed it—okay, it was epic. I don't think I had any more in me, which is a bummer, because if my left hamstring had felt like my right, I'm sure I could have done more.

Here are other positives to being on the other side of the last sixteen weeks. Listening to so much music nearly every day has significantly reduced my stress level, and it occurs to me that dealing with a hamstring injury is not the worst kind of injury to have, since I am able to exercise. It's the injury that prevents you from moving—that's the one you want to avoid.

And training—or sculpting, as Lord Baltimore refers to it—is at a good place. Now Adorable tells me when I have more in me, and although I often disagree, I don't say anything, and I'm trusting him and using all of my focus to get more.

The big change is that every workout, including training, now has added time for rolling and stretching. I start each workout or training on the mat rolling out my calves, quads, IT band, and glutes, and I end each workout or training with six minutes of stretching.

What this means is that I'm at the gym no later than 5:30 a.m. for my early workout, and when I hit the gym in the evening, I stay until 8:00 p.m.. That's an extra hour a day, but both the rolling and the stretching are critical, and I'm noticing the difference.

For cardio, I'm doing three miles on the recumbent bike (resistance set at 5, maintaining 70 RPM); 40 minutes on the elliptical (10 cross ramp—or incline—and resistance at 6); five minutes on the arm bike (set at 3) maintaining 70 RPM, and one mile on the treadmill (between 4.6–5 MPH) before stretching.

I've been baking Apricot Power Bars from a Paleo recipe my sister Phyllis sent me that are absolutely fantastic. I resisted the temptation to swap out almonds for pecans, and I'm so glad I followed the recipe exactly. These are the most awesome power bars to have about an hour before a workout. Try them:

APRICOT POWER BARS

Ingredients

1 cup dried apricots

2 cups pecans

2 large eggs

¼ tsp. sea salt

1 Tbsp. vanilla extract

½ cup dark chocolate chips

Instructions

1. Place apricots and pecans in a food processor and pulse until they are the texture of coarse gravel

2. Pulse in eggs, salt, and vanilla until mixture forms a ball

3. Remove mixture from food processor and work in chocolate chips

4. Place mixture in a greased 9 x 9-inch baking dish

5. Bake for 25 minutes at 350 degrees Fahrenheit

6. Cool and serve.

***

🎵 PLAYLIST HIGHLIGHTS

When I was in Minneapolis, I went to the opening of Christopher Durang's *Vanya and Sonia and Masha and Spike* at the Guthrie, where Adin was assistant directing. Guthrie opening nights are famous for their DJ parties, and I enjoyed dancing to a brilliant mix. I've put together what I'm now calling my Guthrie playlist, which includes what I remember from the party as well as what Adin introduced me to during the marathon drive to Chicago and then home.

Suit & Tie – Justin Timberlake and Jay Z

I Just Wanna Love U (Jay Z)

The Safety Dance – Men Without Hats

Blurred Lines – Robin Thicke

Billie Jean – Michael Jackson

Sing – Ed Sheeran

Dynamite – Talo Cruz

Funkytown – Lipps Inc

Fancy – Iggy Azalea

Shoop – Salt-n-Pepa

Love on Top – Beyoncé

It Wasn't Me – Shaggy (OMG—listen to this one! So hysterical!)

Right Round – Flo Rida

We Sink – Chvrches

Zombie – The Cranberries

Ooh La La – Goldfrapp

Pieces of the People We Love – The Rapture

Dance with Me Tonight – Olly Murs

Summer – Calvin Harris (Totally love this.)

Burn – Ellie Goulding

Deezy Daisy – Portland

Day 141, August 17, 2014

> *"Everybody's got a little piece of someone they hide."*
> —The Rapture, "Pieces of the People We Love"

Now, when people see me for the first time in a few years, they study my face to try to figure out what's different. I don't say anything, I simply smile and then maybe say something like, "Is it my hair?"

People don't want to ask you if you've lost weight or if you've been working out because they don't want you to think they are suggesting you were fat or out of shape before.

"I've been getting fit."

"Oh, I can see it in your face."

This is the fun part of getting in shape, but it's also the most important part—letting your face show how you feel.

Earlier in the week, I was fascinated by a piece in the *New York Times* about young Muslim women blogging about hijab fashion. Only a few years ago, I wrote about a cutting-it-close-to-the-edge exhibit that made me worried for the artists, who used images of the veil to explore identity and culture, working predominantly outside Iran but not necessarily in the United States. While some Muslim artists used the veil to explore tensions between what can be seen and what is hidden by the scarf, other artists, including female artists, used images of the veil to explore women's role in culture and society.

It's like a century has passed as I look at the works featured in the 2009 exhibit now and join the other 900,000 Instagram followers of ascia_akf, who posts fashionable photos of herself wearing a hijab. What strikes me about twenty-four-year-old Ascia Sarrha's pics is her expression, her smile, which conveys confidence, poise, yet possibly a lightness of being. I think Ascia may represent a whole collection of young Muslim women (and men) who believe women can be modest without being invisible, and that they can be educated and take part in popular culture.

These are Western ideas to be sure, but judging by the numbers, definitely a trend. I looked at all of the bloggers cited in the *New York Times* article, and they all seem to wear that same smile. It seems these women wear health on their faces.

I know I've been using the word "epic" a lot lately, but don't kill me if I use it again here. Look at the Instagram photos yourself. Muslim women taking (healthy) photos of themselves and using social media to post them online is unquestionably epic.

***

The last few weeks have been rough for me and for members of the Belkin family. First, we lost my cousin Stanley Kramer, who died in his home in Florida shortly after being released from the hospital. Then on Saturday, August 9, my uncle Stanley Belkin, my father's brother, died in his sleep after returning from Stanley Kramer's funeral and enjoying a stylish lunch at an upscale sushi restaurant in Manhattan with my cousin Arthur Belkin and his son, Jonah Belkin.

Both Stanleys had great enthusiasm for food (Stanley Kramer was a world-class chef) and the other finer things in life, and they were both generous with their love and loyalty to family. When I was at Vassar, I used to stop in at the Oyster Bar in Grand Central Station before catching the Long Island Railroad at Penn Station, and Stanley would come out of the kitchen in his chef's hat and sit with me for a few minutes to make sure I had ordered the best seafood on the menu.

I was talking about this with Stanley's son Jonathan Kramer at the *shiva* at my house on Thursday for my uncle Stanley, and Jonathan reminded me that his father had also been the head chef at the trendy and very hip Thursdays restaurant during the Studio 54 days. He then showed me the picture he had taken on his phone flying into Newark Airport, where the Oyster Bar has a spot opposite Jonathan's arrival gate. Freaky!

So much of what seems important to us day after day appears like a blur when we're at a funeral and looking back. Both Stanleys took hold of each day and grabbed what was good, and that's something the rest of us can feel happy about and continue to embrace in our own lives.

***

It was completely random that my sister Phyllis and her husband, Josh Sessler, were visiting us from New York over the weekend of August 9 and that all of us were in Bethesda exercising in one way or another. My parents, Harriet and Len, were walking on the Capital Crescent Trail while I was running on the trail, Phyllis was at Equinox taking a yoga class, and Lord Baltimore and Josh were taking the Metabolic Effect class at Bethesda Sport and Health when Len got the call.

We spent the rest of the day in my kitchen, making our plans to travel to Yonkers for the funeral. During our many conversations, Josh, another world-class chef, turned me on to a fabulous new band: Clean Bandit. He told me Sofie, Josh's daughter and my niece, had discovered them before they were published on iTunes—she's got a knack. I've been listening to their (first) new album ever since. Some tracks are as good for working out as they are for hosting a dinner party (not easy to do). The band members are apparently classically trained musicians, so that's where the Mozart references come in.

While I was in Westchester for the funeral, I worked out at the Equinox in Armonk (major shout out to that place— fantastic and just as friendly as the Bethesda Equinox). I also joined Phyllis at the Saw Mill Club, where she belongs, and was blown away by the genius "Cardio Cinema." Why didn't I think of that? And now I'm wondering if airlines could offer a spot on a treadmill or elliptical instead of a seat for a two-hour flight.

🎵 PLAYLIST HIGHLIGHTS

Mozart's House – Clean Bandit

Extraordinary – Clean Bandit

Come Over – Clean Bandit (Best track on the album, I think.)

Outro Movement III – Clean Bandit

Thinking About You – Calvin Harris

Somewhereinamerica – Jay Z (I completely love him.)

Pieces of the People We Love – The Rapture (Kind of a theme song these days.)

Day 167, September 12, 2014

> *"I hear a wind/whistling air/whispering in my ear."*
> —B52s, "Roam"

Just before going into a meeting with a person I had never met where the stakes were high, I closed my office door and listened to a little 50 Cent. That's not how I would have prepared for a meeting a few weeks ago, but after coming across a recent Kellogg School of Management study that followed the positive effects of listening to hip-hop music in *Complex Magazine*, I thought I'd give the approach a try. The original article, "Pump Up the Jams and Feel Powerful," was published in the August 4, 2014, edition of *Kellogg Insight*.

I'm not sure how the meeting went, but I remained upbeat throughout the conversation and maybe even a little empowered. I hope my positive energy rubbed off on the other person, because I appreciate it when I'm the recipient of a dose of good old rocky mountain high.

The Kellogg researchers asked whether listening to the right kind of music—even in the background—could make us feel more powerful and in control.

I'm continuing to experiment with listening to podcasts or watching the morning news while I'm on the treadmill, but after a few minutes, I'm back to plugging into my music. There are tons of studies about how music affects both body and mind during exercise. Depending on what you're listening to, music basically distracts us from pain and exhaustion, pumps up our mood, and according to some scientists, can even promote metabolic efficiency.

So I did some reading about this. A 2013 *Scientific American* article quoted sport psychologist Costas Karageorghis of Brunel University in London saying music is a "type of legal performance-enhancing drug."

It's not just about rhythm or beat—it's also about having an emotional connection to a piece of music that triggers a significant (good) memory. I think that's why I've been instinctively turning to my oldies playlists, especially when I'm wondering how much more I've got in me. Seriously, I've been listening to Rod Stewart and R.E.M. nearly every day for weeks, and I can't even tell you if I like their songs, but they absolutely bring back positive memories.

For hip-hop, although I'm always searching for the latest songs and artists, I naturally gravitate to the mid-2000s, because those were the songs Adin and Mia and their friends were playing at their bar and bat mitzvahs, and thus began my love affair with 50 Cent, the Black Eyed Peas, and Terror Squad.

***

So where am I with my goals this month to burn more calories and crush my lower abs? I'm cross-training (impressed?)— running (3 miles) and swimming (30–45 minutes)—and coordinating core, upper-body, and lower body work with

Adorable with work on my own. I'm foam rolling like it's my job, and stretching like crazy after workouts.

Really Smart is adding "load" to my hamstring strengthening exercises, which along with the dry needling is starting to make a difference. She keeps reminding me that hamstring tears take a long time to heal. So yeah, I'm putting in the time and enduring 25–30 pounds on the sadistic leg curl machine.

My plan is to weigh in next week and to compare my BMI with my numbers on Day 1.

Our trip to Berkeley last week set me back in terms of calorie intake, but everything was healthy and delicious, and I'm not going to dwell on it.

It was so great to travel to California with D.C. friends Evelyn and Scott Schreiber and to experience Calshakes through their newbie eyes. As in, really? Are we watching Shakespeare in the hills of Orinda in forty-degree weather wrapped in blankets and parkas?

We also had the chance to catch up with old friends Joe and Terri Tiffany, the original California girl and one of the fittest women I know, who by the way braved the chill in summer sandals, and the brilliant Lori Adels and her husband, Mark Lazar.

As for my lower abs, Adorable has got me strengthening my lower back at the same time because these two are apparently connected. Real results may take longer than I want, mostly because my back needs nearly as much work and this does not happen overnight (though wouldn't that be great).

I've finally gotten some good answers from *Runner's World* on what foods to eat before and after workouts, and armed with a little info, I'm enjoying adding sweet potatoes, curry, and saffron to fish recipes. Here's a fish recipe that is perfect:

RUNNER'S WORLD SALMON COCONUT CURRY

Ingredients

2 tsp. canola oil

2 chopped shallots

2 garlic cloves, minced

2 cups chicken broth

14 oz. light coconut milk

2 sweet potatoes, cubed

2 Tbsp. tomato paste

1 Tbsp. minced ginger

1 Tbsp. curry

1 tsp. cumin

¼ tsp. cayenne

¼ tsp. salt

¼ tsp. pepper

1 lb. salmon, skinless and cubed

1½ cups frozen peas

1 lime, juiced

cilantro

Instructions

1. Heat 2 teaspoons canola oil in a pot.

2. Add 2 chopped shallots and 2 minced garlic cloves; heat 2 minutes.

3. Add 2 cups chicken broth, one 14-ounce can light coconut milk, 2 cubed sweet potatoes, 2 tablespoons tomato paste, 1 tablespoon each minced ginger and curry, 1 teaspoon cumin, and ¼ teaspoon each cayenne, salt, and pepper.

4. Boil, reduce heat, and simmer 20 minutes.

5. Add 1 pound of skinless cubed raw salmon, 1½ cups frozen peas, and juice of 1 lime; simmer 5 minutes.

6. Garnish with cilantro.

***

🎵 PLAYLIST HIGHLIGHTS

Some new favorites and oldies that take me to a good place.

Mozart's House – Clean Bandit featuring Love Ssega

Come with Me Now – Kongos

Latch – Disclosure

Pitbull – Timber

Sweet Dreams – Eurythmics

Peace Train – Cat Stevens

Run-Around – Blues Traveler

Maggie May – Rod Stewart

Family Affair – Mary J Blige

Hips Don't Lie – Shakira

Every Breath You Take – The Police

Burning Down the House – Talking Heads

Roam – B52s

Losing My Religion – REM

Miracles – Jefferson Starship

Baby I Love Your Way – Peter Frampton

Island in the Sun – Weezer

Day 174, September 19, 2014

> *"That's the way it is 'cause life's like this."*
> —Avril Lavigne, "Complicated"

They're not everything, but metrics matter.

I weighed in early Friday morning, and there it was right in front of me. Not only have I gained three pounds since my last time on the scale, but Adorable calculated my body fat as 30.7 percent, which although down from 36.9 percent on Day 1, is still considered overweight.

As hard as Adorable and friends and family have tried to pick me up, the reality is I still have 14 pounds to lose, and even then, I would be technically nine pounds overweight.

I just don't see it happening, despite the fact that I believe I have an aggressive exercise regimen and an extremely thoughtful meal plan.

At this point everything is up for discussion, and at Triathlete's suggestion, it might be time to spend some money on consulting a registered dietician. So far, my meals are fueling my workouts, but maybe I can make slight changes to reduce calories without compromising stamina.

The Paleo-clean eating approach to food makes me feel good, however, I wish I'd see some weight loss.

On Saturday I booked a bike to add studio cycling into my cross-training. The Equinox front desk greeter cheerfully suggested I arrive early to get acclimated.

"If you don't have cycling shoes, the teacher can put a 'cage' around your running shoes."

There are two perspectives on running and weight loss that I'm considering carefully. *Runner's World* coaches discourage thinking about weight loss in any significant way, instead focusing on the tangible benefits of building strength and stamina in addition to all of the psychological perks of running.

Weight loss advocates assert that running regularly, even long distances and at a good pace, causes your metabolism to reset and get stuck, preventing meaningful calorie burn. In particular, this group talks about the weight loss advantages of High-Intensity Interval Training (HIIT), short, intense workouts kind of like sprinting and recovering that supposedly improve metabolism and fat burn.

I've been aware of the benefits of HIIT and at times have tried to sprint during my runs, but as soon as I hit somewhere close to 5.5 MPH, my hamstring freaks out and I need to slow it down.

Lately I've been spending 30 minutes on the elliptical later in the evening and setting the machine on weight loss, which is essentially HIIT; and if I visualize my arms doing the work, I'm able to strengthen my hamstring without crossing the line. I only started adding the late evening cardio work this week, so hopefully I'll see some results on the scale in the near future.

I was talking with my sister Ilene Friday morning, and we went over my exercise and food regimen. I told her I wanted to revisit using weights for calorie burn. Even though I'm afraid I might bulk up, apparently every time you work out, and especially with weights, your muscles experience tiny tears and your body uses energy (calories) to repair the damage.

I know I'm simplifying here, but remember I'm an idiot when it comes to this.

"Are you taking ibuprofen or Tylenol?" Ilene asked. "They can block your body's ability to repair the tears and prevent calorie burn."

Really? When my doctor took me off ibuprofen because of my high blood pressure, I started taking extended release Tylenol once a day for osteoarthritis symptoms. Tylenol also helps manage my hamstring pain, which at times is significant. Moving forward, I'm going cold turkey on that red pill too.

🎵 PLAYLIST HIGHLIGHTS

Pure high-energy Friday morning for my two-mile run after my lovely visit with the body fat calculator and before a session with Adorable. Later in the evening, when Triathlete and I were heading to Woolly Mammoth for the *Marie Antoinette* opening, she turned me on to her favorite pick me up number: "Tubthumping," better known as "I get knocked down" by Chumbawamba. Hilarious. If that one doesn't pick you up, nothing will.

In da Club – 50 Cent

Lean Back – Terror Squad

My Humps – Black Eyed Peas (I'm not kidding, I have a new appreciation for this gem.)

I Am the Best – 2NE1

Sabali – Amadou & Mariam

Switch – Will Smith

Club Can't Handle Me – Flo Rida

Disco Inferno – 50 Cent

Let's Ride – Ground Up

ET – Katy Perry featuring Kanye

OMG – Usher

Yeah – Usher

Burn – Meek Mill

212 – Azealea Banks

After Party – Keith Milgaten

Don't Stop the Party – Pitbull

Mozart's House – Clean Bandit

Escape – Kongos (Lyrics worth listening to.)

Day 185, September 30, 2014

> *"Switch me on/turn me up."*
> —Goldfrapp, "Ooh La La"

I'm not so naive as to think professional athletes should have enough endorphins to keep them from hitting women or punching anyone outside a boxing ring or that walking away from an abuser is simple, but I am seriously perplexed at the continuing high rate of intimate partner violence in this country. Statistics published by the National Domestic Violence Hotline are breathtaking:

◊ On average, 24 people per minute are victims of rape, physical violence, or stalking by an intimate partner in the United States—more than 12 million women and men over the course of a year.

◊ Nearly 3 in 10 women (29 percent) and 1 in 10 men (10 percent) in the United States have experienced rape, physical violence, and/or stalking by a partner and report a related impact on their functioning.

What do we have to do to change it up here? I was struck by the athleticism of the actors playing Hermia, Helena, and Titania at Calshakes' production of *A Midsummer Night's Dream* directed by Shana Cooper. I've come to think of this play, along with *Much Ado About Nothing*, as being athletic linguistically, but Cooper's production of *Dream* takes empowering Shakespeare's leading women to a practically muscular level, and it's an image of women I am digging.

I'm not saying muscular women are not victims of domestic violence, but I do think there needs to be a paradigm shift in what empowerment can look, act, and feel like, especially for women.

It's typically my brain that holds me back physically, so what I'm envisioning for myself and possibly for other women is empowerment that comes from a kinetic synchronicity of mind and body of sorts. Like it takes a muscular mind to build a strong body, and a rockin' body fuels a top-notch brain.

Cooper's coming to Woolly Mammoth Theater Company for a two-year directing residency this winter, and I'm looking forward to her visionary work right here in my hometown.

I'm hyper-focused on the connection between emotional and physical health, so you won't be surprised to learn that's the lens I used to study four plays in New York City this weekend.

Traveling with members of the Woolly family, we had what you could call an intense weekend getaway in realism, beginning with *The Wayside Motor Inn*, written by AR Gurney and directed by Lila Neugebauer, who worked with Mia a few years ago on *The Capeman* in Central Park, and ending with the suffocating reality-show rendering of Ingmar Bergman's classic *Scenes from a Marriage* at New York Theatre Workshop directed by Ivo Van Hove.

All of the women in these two shows, in addition to the women in *The Curious Incident of the Dog in the Night-Time* and *Disgraced,* used their physicality to help define their state of mind.

Disgraced, the Pulitzer Prize winning play by Ayad Akhtar, deals with Pakistani-American Amir Kapoor's self-loathing and his relationships with his WASPy wife, Emily, and another couple, Emily's Jewish gallery owner friend Isaac and his wife Jory, Kapoor's African American law colleague.

There are hints of domestic violence early on in the story, but if you looked at any of the characters, you could not imagine it. I don't want to give too much away, but I can say although the three friends are unable to prevent Kapoor's unraveling, and no one is unscathed by his actions, Emily and Jory are empowered by their muscularity of mind and body.

And by Jory's shoes, which, by the way, were a knock out. Someone needs to find out more about those burgundy pumps.

Even without empowerment, it's hard to imagine being resilient without a fit mind and body. I think that's one of the things Michelle Obama's getting at with her Let's Move campaign for young people, especially girls.

***

I'm a grown-up, and I plan to get back on the scale this weekend despite my last disappointing weigh-in. Since then I've added evening cardio workouts and a bonus mile to my weekend runs.

I can tell by the looks of the trainers I see in the gym the mornings before work and in the evenings after work that they are too polite to ask me if I'm crazy.

Yes, I am.

I'm up to four miles, and the last mile is a real push and a mind / body game I play with myself and with Adorable's voice in my head.

You got it. Don't stop.

The first time I ran four miles (after making it through an insane studio cycling class), I slept for nearly five hours. I was as surprised as anyone that I woke up at all, because I was completely smashed.

I'm still processing whether that was a good thing and whether running might not be great for me (my friend Scott Schreiber, a longtime long-distance runner, says running IS bad for you), but I'm addicted now and there's no turning back. Nothing comes close to the natural high, and I'm running with it, so to speak.

***

Without firm Thanksgiving plans, I told Lord Baltimore I had registered for the Turkey Chase 10K in Bethesda, which would be my first race ever.

"We won't be hosting Thanksgiving this year," I said.

"Why not? What time's the race?"

I don't think Lord Baltimore was factoring in the after-race coma.

I've just started to think about training for the Turkey Chase—mostly because the course includes some hills—but my plan is to do a lot of running. I'm cross-training in the pool and on the elliptical and recumbent bike for calorie burn and training with Adorable for everything else, but the bottom line is, if I'm committed to running a 10K, the most important thing for me to be doing right is to run.

I admitted to Adin in an early phone call on my way to work this morning that I'm enjoying swimming. (He knows how much I hated being on a swim team growing up.) It's an efficient workout. I swim hard for 40 minutes, and I'm back at my house getting ready in an hour. And I'm already showered.

Now that I think about it, I made three phone calls during my thirty-minute drive this morning. I'm super awake after swimming. And chatty.

🎵 PLAYLIST HIGHLIGHTS

I'm fine-tuning a Turkey Chase playlist that is carefully orchestrated. No shuffle here and nothing up to chance. Here's what I've got so far.

Morning Has Broken – Cat Stevens

1234 – Feist

Club Can't Handle Me – Flo Rida

Some Nights – Fun.

Ooh La La – Goldfrapp

Coastin' – Zion I & K. Flay

Down with the Trumpets – Rizzle Kicks

Timber – Pitbull

Comme Un Enfant – Yelle

Crazy Kids – Kesha

I Am the Best – 2NE1

Sabali – Amadou & Mariam

Come with Me Now – Kongos (Have you seen the videos of these brothers?)

We Are the One (Ole Ole) – Pitbull (World Cup song—hard not to picture those gorgeous players when you're listening to this.)

212 – Azealia Banks (Absolutely do not try to decipher the words, as they are beyond raunchy.)

Tainted Love – Soft Cell

In da Club – 50 Cent (This is definitely around the time in my run when I need to hear: "Go shorty, it's your birthday.")

Mozart's House – Clean Bandit (On Saturday I played Jay Z's "Holy Grail" at this point, but I'm not 100 percent down with that—still playing with these two slots.)

We Sink – Chvrches

Come Over – Clean Bandit (I heard Jason Derulo's "Talk Dirty" over the weekend, but too explicit.)

Summer – Calvin Harris

It's Raining Men – The Weather Girls (Just cracks me up every time.)

Day 196, October 13, 2014

"I think with my heart and move with my head."
—Kongos, "Come With Me Now"

Since my hamstring tear in June, I've been expending a lot of energy focusing on preventing injury. The reality, though, is when you've let so much time go by between being a slug and a slightly insane fitness maniac, it's a matter of when, not whether.

"The good news is your hips show no wear and tear, no arthritis, and no deterioration," my orthopedist told me late last week after he x-rayed my left hip to rule out a stress fracture.

It was just after completing the rehab on my left hamstring that Really Smart started adding load to my glute and hamstring exercises. I was doing side planks with hip abduction with Really Smart and Adorable, but then I made the ill-advised decision to do these incredibly challenging exercises on my own. My form slipped, and I sustained a tear in my gluteus medius. By the time I limped into the doctor's office, my mind was already processing how I was going to (1) burn calories without my runs and (2) train for the Turkey Chase on November 27.

So yeah, I'm back in the pool.

My doctor gave me a shot of cortisone into the muscle, which now, four days later, feels much better. I'm aware there is some controversy about whether steroids inhibit muscle repair, but since I am unable to take any NSAIDs, I think it was a good call. There's no way the inflammation would have gone down on its own any time soon, and I was having trouble walking down a hallway or up and down stairs. I'm especially tuned in to the fact that steroids can mask the injury, so I've taken running out of the mix for at least two weeks regardless of how good I feel. I have a new prescription for PT that includes key glute-strengthening exercises.

Really Smart has been all about the glutes for a few weeks now. Recently, she sent me an article by Bret Contreras, the "Glute Guy," which I think is worth checking out. He's not a fan of yoga, but he has some important insights about your buttocks being the butt of all of your weaknesses.

I'm serious about making progress in the pool. I broke down and bought a swim watch and was more than a little surprised to learn that I'd only burned 213 calories in 47 minutes of swimming. Armed with this information, I plan to swim differently tomorrow, but I also need to make sure I understand how the watch works, because it's possible I've got the settings messed up.

∗∗∗

I've dropped below 110 pounds, even if it's just slightly below 110. I haven't weighed less than 110 pounds since before I lived in San Francisco, and if you had been in the women's locker room a few hours ago, you would have seen a person with a ridiculously smiley expression on her face.

So, this is after adding evening cardio to my daily workouts and with keen attention to what I am eating. Even Adorable is asking me what I'm eating, which I'm happy about, because I'm saying aloud what I've been keeping to myself for most of the past six months. You know it's a human trait to spin the information that swirls in your head in a way that helps you get through the day, but when you say something to another person out loud, you have to face the music.

After coming home from my swim at around four o'clock, I was hungry, but since I was having dinner with friends at seven, I knew I could not eat anything significant. I'm slow to come to the green smoothie party, but this is one I like a lot. It's not very caloric but keeps you full for at least a few hours. Most of the recipe comes from Nina Manolson, but I've adjusted things according to my own tastes:

BASIC GREEN SMOOTHIE

Ingredients

2 cups green veggies
(I use kale, but you can use spinach and bok choy.)

1 celery stalk

¼ cup parsley

1 cucumber (I use organic, so I leave on the peel.
You can use 2 baby cucumbers.)

1 whole lemon, peeled

1 banana

2 cups water (Sometimes I use coconut water,
but today I forgot.)

Handful of ice cubes

Instructions

Mix everything in the Vitamix.

***

I've been having discussions with friends, including Ripped, about the whole carbohydrates situation, and I'm trying to be conscious of how many carbs and what kind I'm eating and when.

I'm still doing the high-carb thing 30 minutes before heading to the gym at 5:30 a.m.—small glass of freshly squeezed OJ, half a banana, and a cup of coffee. This is a perfect recipe for success for me, whether I'm doing cardio or training with Adorable. I've experimented with skipping this, but I'm back to doing what I know works.

After morning workouts, however, I've eliminated toast or a whole wheat English muffin in favor of a poached egg, roasted sweet potatoes (with cayenne), and half an avocado. I've been roasting up a batch of sweet potatoes and keeping them in the freezer and about four poached eggs in the fridge so I can heat them up quickly in the microwave after getting home from the gym.

***

🎵 PLAYLIST HIGHLIGHTS

My playlists disappeared from my iPhone when I downloaded the latest system software, so I'm in recovery.

Day 207, October 22, 2014

> *"When the going gets tough/the tough get going."*
> —Pitbull, "We Are One"

Now that I'm incorporating (the tiniest bit of) weight training, I'm engaging in insane conversations with Adorable and runner friends on smart ways to get to *failure*.

Let's just say that in my nine-to-five world, getting to failure just doesn't come up.

When Adorable used the phrase for the first time, I wasn't sure if he was testing me to see if I was paying attention or if I had completely zoned out.

He was adding and taking away weights while I was using a weight machine in a purposeful way when he explained the gist behind the pyramid set versus the drop set.

"We're doing many reps with a lighter weight and then gradually adding weight but with fewer reps," he said matter-of-factly.

"That's a pyramid set. In a drop set, we're starting with a higher weight, and once we get to *failure*, we'll continue without resting with a lower weight."

"Are you making this up?"

"Or we could start with a lower weight, as it works the other way around too."

I've been focusing on pushing myself beyond anything close to my comfort zone. But getting to failure?

Getting to failure is a term used in weight training, but it also applies to exercising without weights. For example, when I'm doing regular, standard push-ups, which we added a week ago, the idea is to go until my muscles fail and then immediately drop to my knees and do as many reps as possible.

It takes intelligence to get to failure, Adorable reminded me.

It's a goal.

Without injury.

We are so done with super setting.

**

Friday will be a month out from the Thanksgiving Turkey Chase and three weeks without running, but until the strain in my left gluteus medius and my oblique muscle heals, I'm using the pool and the elliptical for calorie burn and cardio. Really Smart is direct about not running with a weak butt. Her worry is that I'll put additional strain on my knees, and that's never a good idea.

Also, I'm hyper-focused on my form in the pool to ensure I don't twist a certain way and further irritate my oblique. I've added new music to my swim mix, and that's helping me pay attention and not space out. After 40 minutes in the pool, though, I'm only burning a little more than 200 calories, which seems crazy, but swimming is definitely giving me an all-around workout that comes close to running. Since I'm supplementing with the elliptical and the recumbent bike after work, I'm passing the days until I can get back on the treadmill or the trail with a respectable effort.

And I'm using this time to get educated on the science and chemistry of exercise. My running friend Scott Schreiber sent me links to a two-part article on the importance of incorporating long-duration, low-intensity cardio into your regimen. For starters, performance coach Mike Robertson points out the major benefits of this kind of conditioning:

◊ Improved cardiovascular function

◊ Deeper, more restful sleep

◊ Less stress and anxiety

The idea is that there are two essential forms of energy that our body uses to fuel our metabolism—aerobic, or cardio, and anaerobic, which is what the body uses when you're out of air and it switches over to phosphates (ATP adenosine triphosphate and CP creatine phosphate) and glycolytic energy.

We have very limited stores of ATP in our muscles, so we can't count on ATP for more than a few minutes of intense energy. Glycolytic energy uses glucose as a fuel, and when glucose breaks down, one side effect is the production of lactate, which causes muscles to fatigue and hurt (apparently lactate gives you the "burn" sensation).

In aerobic exercise, oxygen fuels our metabolism, and as long as we're pumping air, we can exercise our muscles without fatigue. So it makes sense to try to increase the amount of time we can go without needing to rely on anaerobic energy. Mostly this is because when we go glycolytic, we can only last a few minutes before the burn shuts us down.

Sprinting and weight training are examples of anaerobic exercise (apparently walking uphill and climbing stairs are, too).

Robertson doesn't oppose using the anaerobic energy system. You need it for lifting weights, and for walking up hills and climbing stairs. But the limits of glycolytic energy production are something like one to two minutes, so you hit a wall quickly.

"There are going to be times when you cross over into glycolytic metabolism," Robertson writes. "That's okay. When you want/need to go hard, you need to have that capacity. But if you fail to train the aerobic system effectively, once you go glycolytic, it's as though you can't get out of it."

So this is where Robertson talks about widening your aerobic window so you can extend your aerobic workout before hitting your anaerobic threshold. The key here is lowering your resting heart rate if it's high (yes, mine is), because the aerobic window is the gap between your resting heart rate and your anaerobic threshold. Robertson says widening your aerobic window is a (deceptively simple) two-step process:

1. If resting heart rate is high, work to lower it.

2. Push up, or raise, anaerobic threshold.

There are times when I want to go back to being completely ignorant and focused on athletic fashion, but now that I'm here, it's like there is a hole in my head that needs filling.

***

I was using the horrible back machine a few sessions ago when Adorable suggested I pause for about 10 seconds before completely raising my upper body.

"Let's try this elevator style," he said.

"Elevator style?"

"We're stopping on every floor."

***

I was having a full-out conversation on What's App with my nephew Alex Schild in Phuket when he suggested I check out ladies' kick boxing for added cardio. Alex, a jiujitsu trainer and fighter and founder of Sabai Gi athletic wear, has been living in Thailand for several years. To strengthen his shoulders, which take the biggest hit in jiujitsu, his morning workout now incorporates surfing, especially for the paddling.

Sa-bai style.

Relaxed, feeling good, comfortable.

🎵 PLAYLIST HIGHLIGHTS

In the pool, I've added Hozier after their Saturday Night Live performance, and at Scott Schreiber's suggestion,

I've added Melissa Etheridge to my Turkey Chase Mix, which I'm still finessing.

Morning Has Broken – Cat Stevens (I know, I know, but this song takes me to a great starting place.)

1234 – Feist (Adin choreographed his first Renegade Dance Company piece for Dance Bethesda to this one years ago—way before its current celebrity status on commercial TV.)

Club Can't Handle Me – Flo Rida (You know how I feel about him.)

Some Nights – Fun.

Ooh La La – Goldfrapp

Coastin' – Zion I & K. Flay

Down With The Trumpets – Rizzle Kicks

Timber – Pitbull

Comme un Enfant – Yelle

Crazy Kids – Kesha

I Am the Best – 2NE1 (Adin sent me this one when he was a freshman member of the Disiac Dance Company at Princeton.)

Sabali – Amadou & Mariam

Come With Me Now – Kongos

We Are One – Pitbull (dreamy)

212 – Azealia Banks

Tainted Love – Soft Cell

In Da Club – 50 Cent

We Run the Night – Havana Brown

Pieces of the People We Love – The Rapture

We Sink – Chvrches

Lovers Eyes – Mumford and Sons

Mozart's House – Clean Bandit

A Little Bit of Me – Melissa Etheridge

Take Me to Church – Hozier

Day 214, October 29, 2014

> *"There's an art to life's distractions."*
> —Hozier, "Someone New"

My morning's death notification training at work is still lingering in my brain, and I was having trouble not thinking about it during my (five-mile!!) evening run.

In my nearly ten years at State, I've only made three death notifications—two small plane crashes and one suicide. With both plane crashes, it felt like I did the death notifications twice—the first time to let a family member know his or her loved one's name was on the manifest of a plane that crashed, and the second time, some weeks later, to say that recovery teams had identified the (partial) remains in a remote spot halfway around the world.

Shortly thereafter—in that conversation or one that followed a day or two later—I needed to ask whether the family wanted the partial remains for funeral purposes or to wait until forensics experts had found everything, or at least more. In other words, would a finger be enough.

I remember each of those conversations as if I had them 10 minutes ago. From my end, I remember working hard in the first few minutes of each call to sound compassionate (because that's how I felt), and credible (because that's what I wanted to be).

At the end of her briefing, Rachel E. Kaul, LCSW, CTS, who has delivered more than 300 death notifications in primarily hospital and trauma situations, including in the aftermath of 9/11, talked about self-care and how crucial managing our own emotional and physical well-being is to the death notification process. Among other things, Rachel highlighted:

1. Nutrition;
2. Exercise;
3. Sleep; and
4. Practice gratitude (more on this later).

It struck me that Rachel's use of the word "nutrition" instead of "food" is at the heart of the challenges many of us face in finding the right mix and amount of food to consume.

This is also at the center of what First Lady Michelle Obama is trying to accomplish with her Let's Move initiative, which she has had trouble defending after teenagers in rural New Mexico filled garbage cans with fruits and vegetables from their school lunches and students in Arkansas built pyramid sculptures from snack size containers of apple sauce before dumping them in the trash.

In fact, the First Lady has been taking a lot of heat for the controversial school lunch program, also known as the Dumpster Derby.

There are so many dimensions to how and what we eat— emotional, cultural, aesthetic, financial—but the one that is so often overlooked is food as nutrition, or fuel. When we think about food in that way, we're forced to become attuned eaters, to be increasingly self-aware about the nutrition our bodies need to be physically and emotionally healthy.

I realize all of this is complicated—and made more complicated by politics—but in the end, what the First Lady and nutrition activists are getting at is the clear connection between how kids fuel their bodies and their physical, emotional, and, I would argue, intellectual well-being.

And not just what they (or we) eat, but how much.

Most of the time, I think some of us eat more than enough food. Even if we're eating the good stuff, there's too much going in, and unless we're born with skinny genes, our bodies pick up extra weight practically overnight. I'm under five feet tall, but I've got the grownup appetite and the cultural interest in food of a person nearly twice my size.

***

I haven't been scientific about changing things up since my disappointing weigh-in last month. Because I've made four changes all at the same time, it's impossible to know what I can ease up on if I wanted to and still get results. Here's what's new:

1. After-work cardio (that's in addition to my early morning cardio or training);

2. Weight training (not a lot);

3. Lunchtime walk; and

4. Skipping the mid-morning yogurt and fruit and seriously cutting back on eating bread. (I haven't eliminated bread from my diet, but I've substituted sweet potatoes for my morning toast, which is practically the only time of day when I regularly eat bread, other than good bread at a good restaurant or bakery.)

Something is working, because I'm lighter on my feet. And I know it shows because people are asking me if I'm eating enough food. I am. Most of us do.

***

I told Lord Baltimore I ran nearly three miles on the Capital Crescent Trail on Saturday (my first run in three weeks) and felt great (after icing).

"I'm confused. I thought today was a walk only day!"

"I changed my mind."

Women do that.

***

After shopping at the Bethesda Central Farm Market on Sunday, I made this—utterly perfect. I've adapted it from Eat Yourself Skinny.

═══

ROASTED SWEET POTATO, QUINOA, AND KALE SALAD

Ingredients

For the salad:

2 medium sweet potatoes, unpeeled and cubed

1 Tbsp. olive oil

1 tsp. garlic powder

½ tsp. onion powder

½ tsp. oregano

½ tsp. chili powder

½ cup uncooked quinoa (I use the pre-rinsed kind— otherwise you'll need to rinse it)

3 cups kale or mixed greens

¼ cup pomegranate seeds or dried cranberries or cherries

For the dressing:

1 Tbsp. red wine vinegar

1 Tbsp. apple cider vinegar

2 Tbsp. olive oil

1 tsp. minced shallots

1½ Tbsp. honey

Instructions

1. Preheat oven to 425 degrees Fahrenheit.

2. Toss the sweet potatoes with the olive oil, garlic powder, onion powder, oregano, and chili powder. Spread sweet potatoes on a baking sheet lined with parchment paper and roast in the oven for about 30 minutes.

3. While sweet potatoes are roasting, add a half cup of water to a small saucepan and add quinoa. Bring quinoa to a boil, cover and reduce heat, and simmer for about 13 minutes. Remove from heat, keeping quinoa covered, and allow it to sit for about 5 minutes.

4. Combine kale, quinoa, and pomegranate seeds, or dried cranberries or cherries, in a large bowl and toss with dressing. Fold in roasted sweet potatoes.

PLAYLIST HIGHLIGHTS

I'm still adjusting my Thanksgiving Turkey Chase Mix; I tried it tonight, and so far, I'm happy with it. I'm debating adding in some Grateful Dead after eating at Ripple in Cleveland Park Saturday night.

Morning Has Broken – Cat Stevens

1234 – Feist

Club Can't Handle Me – Flo Rida

Carry On – Fun. (I swapped out Some Nights for this one—I love recalling their unbelievably fantastic full-out *Singin' in the Rain*-style performance of this at the Grammys.)

Ooh La La – Goldfrapp

Coastin' – Zion I & K. Flay

Down With The Trumpets – Rizzle Kicks

Timber – Pitbull

Comme un Enfant – Yelle

Crazy Kids – Kesha

I Am the Best – 2NE1

Sabali – Amadou & Mariam

Come With Me Now – Kongos

We Are One – Pitbull

212 – Azealia Banks

Tainted Love – Soft Cell

In Da Club – 50 Cent

We Run the Night – Havana Brown

Pieces of the People We Love – The Rapture

We Sink – Chvrches

Lovers Eyes – Mumford and Sons

Mozart's House – Clean Bandit

A Little Bit of Me – Melissa Etheridge

Take Me to Church – Hozier

Envy – 116 (featuring Tedashii, Andy Mineo, KB)

Come Over (featuring Stylo G) – Clean Bandit

Faded – Zhu

One Last Time – Ariana Grande

CHAPTER 5 –
I AM A RUNNER

Day 223, November 7, 2014

> *"My legs are fine, after all they are mine."*
> —Fun., "Carry On"

There's something inherently empowering about running or otherwise exercising without real pain. Maybe liberating is a better word to describe the feeling of self-control, but I also know better than to take myself too seriously.

After coming in from a run on the trail on Halloween, I took off my muddy sneakers before stretching on the Equinox training floor and noticed a tiny circle on my sock just below my big toe on my left foot. I was using a PT strap to stretch my hamstrings and moved my head closer to my foot to read what was written inside the circle.

It was an *L*.

My Balega socks have a left and a right?

Then I looked at the right foot, and of course there was an *L* on that one too.

I've been wearing these socks for seven months and had no clue that each $18 pair came with a left and a right foot.

It doesn't take much to make me feel stupid when it comes to all of this.

***

I'll try to describe the feeling I had last Sunday morning when I ran 6.18 miles at an average pace of 11:54.

It was a crisp morning and I was testing out my (genius) Under Armour Cold Gear and (miraculous) Lululemon running gloves. I had mapped out my run so that I would start in Bethesda and run on the Capital Crescent Trail for about 3.5 miles, just into the District of Columbia, and then head back running until I hit six and then walk the remaining mile or so.

The only problem was how cold I got after I started walking and how wet my head was, because I was wearing my San Francisco ski cap instead of a cap with moisture-wicking technology. By the time I was inside the gym locker room after the run, I was shivering.

So this is something I want to think about in terms of the Turkey Chase on November 27. I'm sure it's going to be cold, and although I get heated quickly when I'm moving, I want to be sure I've got what I need to warm up after the race.

I was completely aware of the music I was listening to. I remember where I was in my run with every song, but more importantly I was hyper-tuned in to my breathing and my stride.

Really Smart had advised, for now, against trying to tighten my core when I run. Her thought is that you want to preserve all of your energy for your breathing and let your muscles relax while you run. You can work the crap out of them later, but while you're on the trail, let everything go so that your oxygen can flow in the most efficient way possible.

I mention this because I had been experimenting with sucking in my stomach because I thought that would keep pressure off my lower back and legs.

But on Sunday, I did exactly what Really Smart suggested, and it was like I was under water with a mask and snorkel. You know that quiet and relaxed feeling when you're breathing in and out through a tube and moving weightlessly.

Very cool and awesomely unexpected.

If you can get yourself to a place where you can run somewhat comfortably at a slow pace, I say go for it. The payoff is ridiculously huge.

***

"Everything feeling alright?" Adorable asked me more than usual the other day.

"Do I look like I'm not feeling okay?"

"You look fantastic as always. I'm just checking."

Adorable was trying to balance keeping me injury free so I can run on November 27 with pushing me to hit another (admittedly much harder) milestone.

We're in agreement about cross-training, but he's emphatic about not running—or even swimming—with even the tiniest discomfort.

What ever happened to no pain, no gain?

So, yeah. Who am I?

***

Mia told me she was having trouble visualizing me running.

I have trouble visualizing me running.

***

I was at my friend Amy Schear's birthday party last night where I knew only one other person. The rooms were filled with extremely rock-solid looking women. Amy was stunning, and our friend Maryam Salass—Washington's very own Persian Sofia Vergara—told me she hadn't worked out in three months, but there was no way I could tell, since she looked as smokin' and elegant as ever.

I was having a conversation with one woman—an athlete all her life—and when I told her I'd started paying attention to my health seven months ago, she said she could not picture how I might have looked then.

"You're so fit."

The gorgeous Bethany Umbel was there, and we spent way more time than you can imagine talking about our exercise lives, including our relationships with our trainers.

I'm clearly addicted to Adorable. Bethany has had so many trainers she lumps them into one big scary pile. The woman she's working with now is first-rate and has Bethany at a good place, but we both agreed, whether it's with a male or female trainer, the intimate, one-on-one experience is as bizarre as it is fascinating and astonishingly productive.

My mind tells me at some point I'll be at a place where I can do this without a trainer, but looking around the room last night, I don't know when that will be.

This is working for us, and I see now that I'm on the other side that this is when it gets fun.

🎵 PLAYLIST HIGHLIGHTS

I listened to my Turkey Chase Mix straight through last Sunday, but this weekend my plan is to shuffle the mix, because I've got too many songs and I can only part with a few of them. I added a couple this week when I ran early on Wednesday morning. Here is where I am.

Morning Has Broken – Cat Stevens

1234 – Feist

Club Can't Handle Me – Flo Rida

Carry On – Fun.

Ooh La La – Goldfrapp

Coastin' – Zion I & K. Flay

Down With The Trumpets – Rizzle Kicks

Timber – Pitbull

Comme un Enfant – Yelle

Crazy Kids – Kesha

I Am the Best – 2NE1

Sabali – Amadou & Mariam

Come With Me Now – Kongos

We Are One – Pitbull

212 – Azealia Banks

Tainted Love – Soft Cell

In Da Club – 50 Cent

We Run the Night – Havana Brown

Pieces of the People We Love – The Rapture

We Sink – Chvrches

Lovers Eyes – Mumford and Sons

Mozart's House – Clean Bandit

A Little Bit of Me – Melissa Etheridge

Take Me to Church – Hozier

Come Over (featuring Stylo G) – Clean Bandit

Faded – Zhu

Rhythm of Love – Plain White T's

Run-Around – Blues Traveler

Ripple – Grateful Dead

Day 237, November 21, 2014

> *"Whoa, come with me now."*
> —Kongos, "Come With Me Now"

You know there are those people who are so articulate that it doesn't matter whether they are speaking to you or putting their thoughts in an email. Both Really Smart and Adorable are like that.

It's a good thing for me that I'm working with them, because there's so much information out there, and sometimes it's not so straightforward. I'm starting from scratch and would be completely overwhelmed if I weren't able to rely on them to get it all organized into a plan, even if I sometimes only get every other word.

"Keep strengthening the glutes—gluteus maximus (hip extension and external rotation) and gluteus medius (hip abduction)," Really Smart wrote me in an email. "Both super important muscle groups for runners."

Did my PT just refer to me as a runner?

I've hit some nice milestones in the past eight months, but this one is a favorite. Since I tend to identify as an out of shape woman with a weak butt, I'm diggin' this.

Really Smart sometimes copies Adorable in her emails to me, which is helpful, because she may as well be writing to me in Tamil, and I need him to translate.

"Stretching technique: contract-relax. Hamstrings as an example: stretch one hamstring supine, with knee straight, push down with 20 percent effort to perform isometric contraction. Then you should have a greater ability to gently stretch further."

If you were trying to find the visual here, welcome to my (new) world.

***

It's not enough that I'm losing weight at a ridiculously slow pace, even if I am trimming down and fitting into the clothes in my closet. Now there's research that shows that working out can cause weight gain. Of course, I already know this from first-hand experience, but the study still leaves a lot of unanswered questions, even if the bottom line is that fitness is more important for health than how much a person weighs.

"Those who want to lose weight should weigh themselves every four weeks to keep them on track, while being mindful of diet and other activities."

Ya think?

***

A few days ago, I had to be at work early, so I set my alarm for 4:30 a.m. in order to get to the gym to swim by 5:00 a.m. As I was pulling my stuff out of my bag in the locker room, I realized I did not have my music.

It's a good thing I live five minutes away. I raced home to grab my Waterfi shuffle, but when I was back at the lockers, I could not find my swim cap.

I had paused for a moment to decide whether the gym requires swimmers to wear a cap when my workout friend Robyn Shields asked me what was wrong.

"I forgot my swim cap."

"Here, take my car keys," Robyn offered. "My car's right out front, and my swim bag is on the back seat. You can borrow my cap."

I've been practicing gratitude obsessively since setting out on this journey, but I can't express enough how encircled I feel these days. Some of my emotion is jumpstarted by the constant rush of endorphins, but I also have deep appreciation for the people who steady and steer me.

I'm also simply grateful to be part of this world of people high on endorphins—the swimmers and runners and walkers out there on the trail and at the gym, and the genius engineers who design and manufacture gear that keeps you warm in 37 degrees and your skeleton in one piece during seven miles of pebbly terrain.

So yeah, I'm feeling good and supported, and I'm keeping my focus, but just the same, I am freaked out about participating in my first race on November 27.

Maybe it's because I'm totally green, but everything about the race has me worried.

Aside from trying to keep myself injury free and immune from flu germs, here's some of what is streaking through my brain.

1. Where to stash my waiting-around-in-the-freezing-cold clothes;

2. Getting through the race without making a pit stop (and if I need one, where);

3. On this note, when to stop eating and drinking; and

4. What to eat and drink.

One plus is that Mia, who ran nearly seven miles with me in Central Park last weekend, is registered to run the 10k. She's got a much quicker pace, but she's a great running partner and is happy to hang back with me. She looks good in running clothes, too, and is more than willing to share her youthful mojo.

***

🎵 PLAYLIST HIGHLIGHTS

My Turkey Chase Mix is looking good, but don't judge—I just added LMFAO's "Sexy and I Know It," and it's so dope. Since it was hard to fit in some of my regular cardio workouts this week, I did more walking in the neighborhood than usual and found myself drawn to my original Ladies Night mix with a few later additions.

Us Against the World – Coldplay

Everybody – Ingrid Michaelson

At Last – Eva Cassidy

I'm Yours – Jason Mraz

Somewhere Over the Rainbow – Israel Kamakawiwo'ole

Hello – Tristan Prettyman

Woods – Bon Iver

I Remember – Lauryn Hill

River God – Nichole Nordeman

Rhythm of Love – Plain White Ts

All This Beauty – Weepies

Keep Breathing – Ingrid Michaelson

Set Fire to the Rain – Adele

Somewhere Only We Know – Keane

Flightless Bird – Iron & Wine

Dreams Be Dreams – Jack Johnson

Nighty Night – Jenny Owen Youngs

Happy Ending – Mika

The Con – Tegan and Sara

Little Lion Man – Mumford and Sons

Quelqu'un m'a dit – Carla Bruni

Dog Days Are Over – Florence + the Machine

Day 247, December 1, 2014

"Take it hip to hip, rock it through the wilderness."
—B-52s, "Roam"

Well, that's out of the way.

Thursday's Turkey Chase 10k was so epic it's hard for me to write about it without smiling.

The day started out in such a spectacular way—the air was cold (34 degrees) and crisp but dry, and the sun was bright against a gorgeous blue sky. I benefited from the excellent advice of friends and family who had run races before, and here's a wrap-up of what went down, according to my list of worries:

1. Where to stash my waiting-around-in-the-freezing-cold clothes – *We arrived at around 7:15 a.m., which gave us a little over an hour before the 8:30 start. Parking was plentiful, so we stayed warm in the car until 7:30 and left our coats in the trunk before walking to the staging area. We enjoyed some people-watching from the car:*

    Mia: "I think we might be the most stylish-looking runners so far."

2. Getting through the race without making a pit stop and if I need one, where – *I didn't need it, and Mia pushed through without looking for one. There would*

> *have been a few options once we got to Wisconsin Ave.*
> *if we needed them, but we were good on this.*

3.   On this note, when to stop eating and drinking –
       We were downstairs in the kitchen by 6:00 a.m.

4.   What to eat and drink – *Me: whole banana (usually*
       I have a half, but I decided I needed the extra fuel);
       small glass of freshly squeezed orange juice, cup of
       black coffee; Mia: banana with peanut butter, water.

Adorable had told me to expect a party atmosphere, and he was right. There was a DJ playing dance music that got the nearly 10,000 runners/walkers moving (including me), and then someone (I didn't catch his name) led us in a warm-up just before lining up according to our run times for the "wave" start.

Before we knew it, we were toasty in our Under Armour Cold Gear and practically skipping across the starting line. The course was unbelievably hilly. Mia, who was trying to keep my spirits up, noted as we approached the peak of the first big hill that whatever goes up has to come down. We quickly learned that there was never a real down on this run. By the time we hit the sixth or seventh hill, I looked over at Mia.

"WTF?"

"You got this, Mom."

My glutes were literally on fire by the time we crossed the finish, and I don't think I've ever pushed as hard on a run.

We finished at 1:14:14 with an average pace of 11:57. We were caught up in the momentum of it all and enjoyed the encouragement of bystanders along the route cheering us on. There were runners as far as the eye could see, both in front of us and behind us. Dancing across the finish line we felt a terrific sense of accomplishment.

My sister Phyllis and her family from New York were visiting for Thanksgiving, and along with Lord Baltimore and my father, Len Belkin, they finished the two-mile Turkey Chase fun walk. After the race, we headed back to my house for brunch, where we enjoyed mimosas, Bethesda "flagels," fruit, and generous slices of my favorite chocolate coffee strip from the legendary Baltimore Jewish bakery Parisers.

The whole thing was simply awesome from beginning to end, and I just want to say for the record, if I can do this, anybody can. For proof, it wasn't too long ago that it took me nearly forty-five-minutes on the treadmill to walk a single mile.

**

In setting my fitness goals for December, I'm changing up my regimen in order to progress on strengthening my muscles. Now I'm focusing on:

- ◊ Endurance;
- ◊ Resistance (load);
- ◊ Repetitions;
- ◊ Intensity; and
- ◊ Power (too advanced for now—more about this later).

It was Adorable who first raised the concern of working out two times per day versus one workout where I'm pushing myself. Really Smart agreed that if my workouts are challenging, I need to give my muscles adequate time to recover in order to make progress. For the past few months, it has made sense for me to do two workouts per day, as I've been focusing on calorie burn and discipline; and although I'm still worried about not getting that extra push at the end of the day, for now, this is the way to go.

I chose to explore intensity on Saturday before training with Adorable, where I ran 3.06 miles at an average pace of 8 minutes. This is way faster than my usual 11–12 minute pace, and for much of the time I could feel my heart practically relocate into my throat.

I'm trying to take the same approach in my training sessions—fewer breaks, for example. These are big goals, and it may take me the entire month to come close to any of them, but no one can accuse me of not walking the walk.

🎵 PLAYLIST HIGHLIGHTS

My Turkey Chase Mix was perfect, so of course I'm starting to think about expanding my run mix to go longer distances. Here's what I've got so far, which is heavy on the rock 'n' roll, along with a few additions Adin introduced me to over the Thanksgiving holiday. My niece Sofie's friend Josh stayed with us over the weekend, and I'm into his band's house party music. Check out Otter at bandcamp.com or on Facebook.

Lakehouse – Of Monsters and Men

Open – Regina Spektor

It's Alright Brother – Otter

I Can't Get No Satisfaction – Rolling Stones

Because the Night – Patti Smith

Brandy – Looking Glass

Sunshine of Your Love – Cream

Bad Day – Daniel Powter

Take It Easy – Eagles

Drunken Lullabies – Flogging Molly

How to Save a Life – The Fray

Sugar Magnolia – Grateful Dead

Satellite – Guster

Somebody to Love – Jefferson Airplane

Heaven – Los Lonely Boys

Semi-Charmed Life – Third Eye Blind

Welcome to Paradise – Green Day

We Will Rock You – Queen

Moondance – Van Morrison

Ramblin' Man – Allman Brothers Band

Could You Be Loved – Bob Marley

While My Guitar Gently Weeps – George Harrison

Day 248, December 2, 2014

"One single moment your whole life can turn around."
—The Streets, "Dry Your Eyes"

I crave the endorphin rush, especially in the morning, and it's always an effort fighting off the stress of my commute so I can hold on to that feel-good vibe for as long as possible into the workday.

There are more distracted drivers than ever, and if you took an aerial view of Connecticut Avenue during rush hour, you'd see cars stopped randomly because (1) drivers have their eyes in their laps and haven't noticed that the light has turned green; and (2) the driver behind hasn't noticed that the car in front has missed the light because that driver is also reading and sending texts and emails.

Not to mention sharing the road with bicyclists—many of them my colleagues at State, especially when I turn onto Pennsylvania Avenue in Foggy Bottom. It's a miracle every morning that I haven't struck or otherwise traumatized a person on a bike. (No offense, cyclists, someday I'll join you.)

My point here is that I treasure the morning workout endorphin rush, and I place a high value on protecting it.

My plan for this morning, Day 2 of my new one-workout-per-day regimen, was to do an Adorable-inspired micro triathlon biking session for 10 minutes on the recumbent bike, run two miles on the treadmill, and then swim for 30 minutes before racing to a doctor's appointment to have a growth biopsied.

Even though I managed to do all of this *and* persuade my doctor to use a shaving technique rather than a punch biopsy to avoid needing stitches that would keep me from exercising for ten days, I wasn't able to shake the disturbing article that popped up in my 6:00 a.m. briefing on my NYT mobile app.

The story was at the bottom of the feed, but it grabbed my attention because Adin is a Princeton student (and a member of an Eating Club, although not the one referenced in the article), and what Princeton parent wouldn't welcome Princeton news that doesn't mention meningitis? And in the *New York Times.* But this piece wasn't one a parent—or any woman, if I'm speaking for myself—wants to read.

If the article's headline, "Princeton Eating Club Ousts 2 Officers Over Emails Ridiculing Women," wasn't bad enough, the article referenced related disturbing instances at Wesleyan reported by the *Washington Post.*

And then Adin pointed me to a first-person account from a freshman rape victim at Vassar who failed to get the support she needed from the college.

Setting aside the alarming lack of cultural awareness evident in the issues raised by the Princeton emails, here is where I'm particularly stuck: If you leave your wallet unattended on a Starbucks counter while you put milk and sugar in your coffee and someone steals it, it's definitely your fault for not holding on to your stuff, but it's still a crime to steal a person's wallet.

While you were the idiot in this scenario, the thief, if caught, especially on video, can be tried and convicted and sentenced for committing a crime.

In the case of the Vassar freshman woman, who blacked out and vomited multiple times after consuming the vodka she carried in her own water bottle at a party and then awoke as she was being raped by the sober male roommate of a friend, the woman is the idiot, but the person who committed the criminal act is the sober guy.

It's as simple as that.

There can never be anything consensual about sex with a person who's drunk or high on drugs. I don't know what went down at the Vassar administrative proceedings or why the freshman woman did not pursue criminal charges in Poughkeepsie, but that's not the only reason why I'm so deeply disturbed by the increasing number of reported instances of rape and sexual assault on college campuses typically associated with crazy excessive drinking and by the complete lack of assistance and support for rape victims, even if they themselves made unbelievably poor decisions.

A victim is a victim, even if the victim is stupid; and a person who commits rape or otherwise sexually assaults another person is a criminal and should be held legally responsible for any criminal act.

Simple?

I know college campuses are trying to figure this out, and many, including Princeton, are holding all students accountable for their safety by imposing zero tolerance policies for sexual assault, but what eludes me (among a lot of other issues) is the underlying sexual dysfunction of teenagers and young adults especially.

We thought we had made progress as women (and now mothers) who memorized *Our Bodies, Ourselves,* and we attempted to raise boys sensitized to sexual equality and girls empowered to enjoy healthy sexual relations and to take responsibility for both sexual wellness and birth control.

But we're still dealing with a culture of boys who should be punished for behaving criminally but are instead getting away with behaving badly. This is because of institutionalized sexism and a tradition of hegemony at universities in which women and individuals who do not identify as heterosexual white men are still treated as outsiders, and as threats to a system that often protects a small and elite class of citizens.

Did this sober college-age male think he was having sex with a comatose woman who had vomited multiple times on herself and in her bed? This is aggression and violence. And power. Not sex.

And in a conversation about this with Mia, she points out there is a long history in our culture of women being held back because they don't own their choices. They feel guilty about having sexual desires, so getting drunk removes some of that.

Nevertheless, men and women involved in nonconsensual sex are ultimately engaging in unhealthy sexual relationships that have an arguably negative impact on how they conduct their sexual lives in the future.

I don't know what to say or understand about how far we've come in terms of our sexual health. We need to do better as parents and teachers and coaches and medical professionals and friends, because it's obvious we're missing a great deal about the teenage brain, and we're not getting through to our young adult children.

I'm glad social media is around to bring these incidents out in the open because I know kids are talking about them. But I wish I had more wisdom to offer here, and that disturbs me maybe as much as anything else.

***

Since I live five minutes from the gym, I don't usually bring my work clothes with me in the morning. I'll shower and wash my hair after a swim, but I'll head home to have breakfast, walk the dog, and get dressed.

I was packing in a more intense workout than usual and needed to get to the doctor's office before work, so I took a suit I hadn't worn in a while to the gym and was pleasantly surprised when I needed to keep my trousers up by tightening my belt. The jacket still fits comfortably, but the pants need to be taken in.

I haven't weighed myself in a fairly long time, but I'm going to plan to do it on Friday morning. I hope the numbers on the scale match up with how loosely my clothes are fitting.

🎵 PLAYLIST HIGHLIGHTS

I listened to my oldies mix and my hip-hop mix on the treadmill (after reading my morning news briefing on the recumbent bike) and in the pool. Here's what stands out from the morning:

The Boogie That Be – Black Eyed Peas

Dry Your Eyes – The Streets

Mockingbird – Eminem

Sunshine – Mos Def

We Be Burnin' – Sean Paul

OMG – Usher

Lean Back – Terror Squad

Talk about a Girl – Charizma & Peanut Butter Wolf

Ooh Kill 'Em – Meek Mill

Family Affair – Mary J. Blige

Empire State of Mind – Jay Z featuring Alicia Keys

Silver Screen – Felix da Housecat

Every Breath You Take – The Police

Fast Car – Tracy Chapman

Pale Blue Eyes – The Velvet Underground

Day 257, December 11, 2014

> *"Don't stop the party."*
> —Pitbull, "Don't Stop the Party"

I'm always looking for the contrast in things, because I think that's where you find the excitement. You know when you see Rodin's *The Thinker*, and of course it weighs a ton, but at any moment that guy could step away from his pose and whack his head, wishing he'd had a V8. Or any of Michelangelo's sculptures of figures draped in "fabric" that are far from light and slippery.

Or when a rail-thin person can blast through 20 push-ups. It's the contrast of little and big that is super interesting, because you just don't expect it.

And I love it when I walk away from live theater shaking my head and wondering, sometimes audibly, what was that?

That's how I felt last night when I saw the Old Trout Puppet Workshop's production of *Famous Puppet Death Scenes* at Woolly Mammoth. In an interview, the Old Trout artists themselves mentioned their fascination with puppets straddling between the living and the dead, which they said inspires an existential focus on themes that are weighty for a puppet show.

In other words, it's the contrast of using puppetry, which we associate with whimsy, to approach weighty issues of death, happiness, and love.

"But a central driving question in our work has very little to do with puppets per se. It's this: what are we all doing in this room together right now? What could we possibly be hoping to accomplish? There's something so peculiar and wonderful about the bare fact of a bunch of otherwise sane people gathered together to pretend that a block of wood has hopes and dreams and terrors.

"Are we here just to understand each other better, or is there something deeper at work; something we don't entirely understand just yet; something in our bones that isn't so easily described? With each show, we attempt in some way to answer, or maybe just ask, those questions."

—*The Old Trout Puppet Workshop*

***

I went to my first holiday open house of the season last weekend and took pleasure in getting ready in five minutes. All I needed to do was grab something festive from my closet and put it on. For the first time in years, everything in there fits; some things a little loosely, although I'm fine with that, too.

So here are the two things I want to mention about holiday parties:

1.   How you feel; and

2.   How you look.

I would say these are one and the same, because most of the time, how you feel is how you look.

Not a stroke of genius but so clutch this time of year.

Because holiday parties—whether they are work or social— are not really parties. Not the way a birthday party is a party or a Super Bowl party is a party, or even how New Year's Eve is a party. Holiday parties are networking events to remind you at least once a year that you are alive and a social being, whether at work or in the neighborhood, and how much you need to put yourself out there.

Working the holiday party has never been more essential because in our day-to-day, we are often tied to our computers and smartphones and barely step outside our cubes to talk with our colleagues. We have meetings via digital video conference or teleconference and telework in our PJs. Yeah, we're all spokes in the wheels that make the world go round, but in reality, we're all far removed from the hub.

The payoff of getting my priorities straight and focusing on me has always been about feeling good, but it's just not possible to disentangle the feeling of well-being from looking good.

It's great when people who haven't seen me in a year tell me I look good, but it's even better socializing without being self-conscious, tugging at my waistband, or otherwise fixing something that's not right on my body; or wrapping a pashmina around my shoulders and torso, no matter how stylish or well-made.

Deep in conversation with one of Lord Baltimore's former colleagues, I was enjoying catching up with her and hearing about her children and her hobbies. We were well into moving from subject to subject when she looked at me and said out of nowhere, "You look so amazingly awesome."

She was noticing that I feel so awesomely physically good in contrast to how fatigued and out of shape and crappy I felt last year at this time.

And it's the contrast of how I felt last year at this time that's giving me the energy and the desire to get out there and socialize. I'm a mega-extrovert, but even extroverts need the right mojo to work a holiday party.

Karen Burns, whose Working Girl blog often untangles the common workplace mess, has some great rules to live by at both office and neighbor holiday parties. I've selected my favorites here and added some of my own bits of wisdom. You can read the full blog post at: http://jobs.seattletimes. com/careercenter/work-life-blog/working-the-workplace-holiday-party/

⬧ Dress conservatively. Do you really want to be remembered as the person who wore a Santa hat with flashing twinkly lights?

⬧ Don't drink alcohol. Or don't drink too much alcohol. You know the difference.

◊ Circulate. Don't spend more than 10 minutes with any one person or group.

◊ Don't be the first to leave. You do not want to give the impression that you're just putting in an appearance.

◊ Keep your conversation positive and upbeat. It's okay to discuss some business or politics, but try to keep it to a minimum.

◊ Don't pig out at the food table. Moderation is good for your image as well as your waistline. Also, only choose food that you can eat easily and without making a mess.

◊ Chat with your boss. This is your chance to get to know him or her on a personal level.

◊ Don't do anything memorable. If a week later, people are still talking about something you did or said, that is almost always a bad thing.

◊ Don't wait to be properly introduced. It may never happen! Take the initiative and introduce yourself.

◊ Finally, remember that while they may call it a party, you are not truly off duty whether in the neighborhood or at the office.

There's a lot out there on how to get the most out of holiday parties, including going armed with a 60-second public service announcement about you. I'm not crazy about that idea, especially as an extrovert who is already trying hard not to talk too much, but I do want to make a strong case for putting in the effort to do what you need to do to feel good.

No matter how much time you put into finding the perfect holiday outfit, I don't think you can do any better for yourself than arriving fit and light on your feet.

***

At Adorable's suggestion, I packed a handful of gummy bears in my pocket and ate a few every mile. I also took some Swedish Fish with me, which although they taste great, tend to stick to your teeth (thus preserving the flavor in your mouth for longer and, as Adorable pointed out, giving you something to focus on). But they also have the potential to get caught in your throat (thus choking you and putting an end to your run). I know some people have a lot of success with high-energy products, and I may try one next time.

PLAYLIST HIGHLIGHTS

On Sunday I did an eight-mile run from Bethesda to Georgetown on the Capital Crescent Trail, stopping to use the surprisingly convenient and clean restrooms at Fletcher's Cove (formerly Fletcher's Boat House), and put together a Long Run Mix that I'm still tweaking.

My Long Run Mix:

I put it on shuffle, so I didn't get to hear every song

Feel Good Inc – Gorillaz

Fancy – Iggy Azalea

Hopeless Wanderer – Mumford and Sons

Switch – Will Smith

Reflektor – Arcade Fire

Paper Planes – M.I.A.

Happy – Pharrell Williams

Rhythm of Love – Plain White T's

Home – Edward Sharpe and the Magnetic Zeros

Club Can't Handle Me Now – Flo Rida

Ooh La La – Goldfrapp

Timber – Pitbull

Comme Un Enfant – Yelle

Come with Me Now – Kongos

212 – Azealia Banks

We Run the Night – Havana Brown

Mozart's House – Clean Bandit

Lakehouse – Of Monsters and Men

Don't Stop Believin' – Journey

While My Guitar Gently Weeps – George Harrison

God Only Knows – Bryan Adams (I love, love, love Bryan Adam's new album—I could listen to this song on repeat for probably an hour.)

The Safety Dance – Men Without Hats

Funkytown – Lipps

Summer – Calvin Harris

SexyBack – Justin Timberlake

Smack That – Akon

Electric Avenue – Eddy Grant

Don't Matter – Akon

Kingston Town – UB40

Redemption Song – Bob Marley

Saturday in the Park – Chicago

Time After Time – Cyndi Lauper

Closer to the Sun – Slightly Stoopid

The Con – Tegan and Sara

Dog Days Are Over – Florence + the Machine

Count on Me – Bruno Mars

I'll Stand by You – Pretenders (Forgot how great this one is, especially live.)

Day 262, December 16, 2014

"I ain't too proud to say."
—Bryan Adams, "You've Been a Friend to Me"

Triathlete and I were at Chalin's eating Chinese lettuce wraps for lunch last week when I told her Adorable was leaving Equinox to pursue academic studies full time.

"OMG, he's breaking up with you!"

"This isn't funny."

"This is good for you."

"It sucks."

"Read Elisabeth Kubler-Ross. You're fine."

As in the five stages of grief?

"You're in denial."

"I'm happy for him, but does this have to happen now? I'm not where I need to be."

"And you're angry."

"I'm completely pissed off."

"You'll make the most of the few sessions you have left. Then you'll be depressed."

"I'm already depressed."

"But you know you'll be absolutely okay. I'll run with you. You'll be fine."

"I'm not going to be fine."

"You're going to be totally awesome."

"Okay fine. I'll be fine. When will you run with me?"

Ripped texted me after Adorable called her to break up with her, too.

"So now we're Rue-less."

Ripped is more advanced, as she's been working out for years and benefited from having a kickass trainer when she worked downtown. But she told me she had learned a lot from Adorable. And so did our Vassar classmate Liz Nagy and her husband, Chris Masters. Both of them had started training with him only three or four months ago.

He has cross-trained our minds and set us up with some good habits.

Here's what I want to say about this:

It's actually okay.

Look what Adorable has accomplished with me.

Let's recap Day 1, where it took me 45 minutes to walk a mile on the treadmill. I was out of shape, overweight, and embarrassed to be walking onto the gym training floor.

Today I am registered to run in the D.C. Rock 'n' Roll Half Marathon, and last Sunday I ran eight miles on the Capital Crescent Trail.

I am a runner.

It was Adorable who explained to me that "heat gear" is stuff you wear to keep cool and "cold gear" keeps you warm. You put weights down as you pull up, and failure is a goal.

Adorable is moving on to a challenging next chapter pursuing physical therapy, where he will have the opportunity to make a real difference in the lives of many more people.

I'm moving on to my next chapter, too. Despite the crazy difference in our ages, Adorable has managed to teach me fundamentals I had never spent two minutes thinking about.

1. This journey is about me. He taught me how to have a relationship with myself. How to prioritize my focus.

2. He's made me passionate about fitness but smart. I'm making intelligent choices about cross-training, when to run, how far, how fast.

3. Adorable is all about results and setting goals. He's got me hyper-focused on making sure my goals are specific, measurable, attainable, realistic, timely. SMART.

4. Adorable got me to my edge and on the other side. I'm not able to do this on my own, but it's my No. 1 goal. I'm not going anywhere on this journey if I can't achieve this one.

Ultimately, in my relationship with Adorable, it's never been about how I look. The endgame has always been about how I feel. That's a part of him that will stay with me and help me get comfortable with another trainer.

We're thrilled that Adorable is following his passion, and all of us will move on to another trainer extraordinaire.

We're okay with this, but we know it won't be the same.

He was that good.

And I ain't too proud to say he was a friend to me.

Just saying.

***

🎵 PLAYLIST HIGHLIGHTS

One of my favorite things about the holidays is Christmas music. As a Jewish girl from Long Island, I know how strangely that rolls off the tongue, but readers who know me well get this about me. Here's what I'm shuffling in the pool this week:

Jingle Bells (Bass) – Basshunter

Have Yourself a Merry Little Christmas – James Taylor

White Christmas – Otis Redding

Peace on Earth/Little Drummer Boy – Bing Crosby & David Bowie (The 4-minute version has their conversation at the start—precious.)

Baby, It's Cold Outside – Lady Antebellum

Amazing Grace – Human Nature

Angels We Have Heard on High – Cast of Scarlet Pimpernel (From *Carols for a Cure 1999*—you can definitely listen to the entire CD straight through—the best *Carols for a Cure* by far.)

Merry Christmas, Baby – Cee Lo Green and Rod Stewart

Little Drummer Girl – Alicia Keys

We Three Kings – Beach Boys

Panis Angelicus – Jewel

Run Rudolph Run – Bryan Adams

Silent Night – Stevie Nicks

Let It Go – Pentatonix (My colleague Chris Abrams sent me a link to the latest from Pentatonix when he heard about my interest in Christmas music—brilliant.)

Nutcracker – Dance of the Sugar Plum Fairy

North Pole Express – Jon Schmidt

Fairy Tale of New York – The Pogues

Do You Hear What I Hear – Whitney Houston

O Come, O Come, Emmanuel – Sugarland

Please Come Home for Christmas – The Eagles

The Chipmunk Song – The Chipmunks

O Holy Night – Glee Cast

Day 277, December 31, 2014

"I won't rest until I know I'll have it all."

—From the Pippin soundtrack, "Corner of the Sky," performed by Matthew James Thomas

After nine months of disciplined focus, I am closing out 2014 and entering the New Year with some reflections.

There isn't anything magical about what I set to accomplish. But here's what is simple: If I can do this, you can, too.

Cross-training: I did a 10-mile run with the MCRRC on Sunday, and as I was getting to know the other runners in my pace group, I was amazed to learn that few of them cross-train. They simply run once or twice a week. Most of them for years. It's crazy to think about how much cross-training I do just so I can run. Crazy, but so worth it.

I've finally gotten to a place where I can use exercise to cross-train my mind. Especially on long runs, I am able to think creatively about issues at work as my brain takes me to the most interesting places. This is new and very welcome.

Attuned eating: It was a paradigm shift when I chose to use food as fuel for my workouts. I've removed all processed foods (except for the clutch gummy bears and Swedish Fish that I use to refuel on my long runs) and rely on super foods. I'm eating as many calories as I need, and surprisingly, I am not hungry. I eat one to two hours before a workout and follow the guidelines in *Runner's World* for what to eat before and after exercise.

I don't succumb to peer pressure when I'm surrounded by French fries or desserts. I've had plenty of potatoes and donuts to last me the rest of my life, and if I ever feel the desire to have them again, I will—in moderation.

It was my sister-in-law Susan Walker who quoted Kate Moss at dinner a few days ago. "Nothing tastes as good as skinny feels." Susan and our sister-in-law Nicole Upton have been on this journey together, and all three of us have seen amazing results.

Supplements: I take these daily and have found the best sources to be USANA and HUM Nutrition. Before you can order from HUM, you have to complete an online questionnaire that is reviewed by a dietician who then makes recommendations. I'm taking vitamin E, calcium with D3, turmeric and phyto-polyphenols, vitamin C and bioflavonoids, probiotics, and a 7-keto, green tea leaf, and chromium combination.

Research: I read everything I can find on nutrition, avoiding and recovering from injury, gear, and inspiration. I'm interested in anything related to fitness and have learned how to sift through the muck to get to the good stuff. I even googled my emotional dependency on Adorable and found comfort in learning how common it is for people to become attached to a great trainer. (One friend told me she was so traumatized after losing her trainer that she hasn't been able to try another one, and it has been nearly a year.)

I subscribe to *Runner's World, Women's Running, Cooking Light,* and *Eating Well,* and my favorite blogs are Robertson's Training Systems and the extremely well written blog published by Equinox. I don't think you have to be a member to subscribe to this one, and in addition to terrific articles, the blog also serves as an aggregator of newsworthy items in the section at the end that highlights what the blog editors have been reading.

Personal training: I was slow to come to this party. True, I had the benefit of Adorable, an altogether out of this world and spectacular trainer, but as I've moved on to Shoubry Sos, my new, buff trainer at Equinox Bethesda, I accept I am only going to get out of this what I put in. After my second session with Buff, I can tell he is observing me carefully to see what I'm about. I get how hard it is for people—young and old—to take me seriously in terms of my fitness goals. (Think young buck trainer and old school orthopedic surgeon.) So I'm giving this new relationship some time to develop.

Physical therapy: Maybe if I had been an athlete at some point in my life, I wouldn't find everything Really Smart tells me so fascinating. I've learned so much from her and Adorable—they are like the Mod Squad of fitness gurus—and I'm glad I have both of them in my life. If your doctor prescribes PT, take it seriously, and do your exercises. They work.

Sleep: I'm strategic about my need to get seven or eight hours of sleep every night. That means I'm in bed by 9:00 p.m. if my alarm is set for 5:00 a.m. Whatever sleep issues I had a year ago are completely gone. I fall asleep easily and wake up feeling rested and energized.

That also means I'm not doing much in my life, especially during the week, other than working out, going to work, and shopping and meal preparation. I only have time for minimal reading for pleasure, very few social events during the week, and even limited conversation at home. Maybe this is the part that requires the most support from family, because if Lord Baltimore made me feel guilty about getting my sleep, I think that would be hard to work through.

Gear: For pants, I'm still convinced my Lululemons are the best. I'm wearing Nike Dri-FIT tanks in the gym as a base layer with Under Armour HeatGear long sleeve crew tops. For running outside, I cannot say enough awesome things about Under Armour's ColdGear. Even in 34 degrees, all I need is the ColdGear fitted long sleeve crew under the ColdGear UA qualifier half zip.

For swimming, I'm using the Garmin Swim Watch (low tech and affordable), and I transfer the data to my MapMyFitness app, which keeps track of all of my workouts, including my runs with MapMyRun. I pay about $5/month for MapMyRun's audio coaching, which I think is worth it.

I've experimented with different gloves and hats, and lately I'm preferring North Face running gloves and an Under Armour hat. The key is to be sure everything you wear fits snugly in order to keep you warm, and that it has Dri-FIT technology so that nothing gets wet. (I'm absolutely amazed at this aspect of today's gear.)

No matter what running store I visit, everyone puts me in a Brooks shoe, so I'm sticking with that. At least until you know what works for you, go to a running store that can analyze your feet and your gait and get you fitted correctly.

In the pool, I use my Waterfi waterproof iPod shuffle to listen to music—I'm not sure what else is out there.

It was Adorable's suggestion to keep spare gear in the car so I can go for a run if I need to blow off steam. And I keep an extra pair of Brooks under my desk at work for times when I can fit in a lunchtime walk.

My relationship with the scale: Today I weigh 107 pounds That's a total loss of 14 pounds, which honestly seems pathetic. But in terms of results, my body is half of what it was on Day 1. So I am done with my obsession with the scale. I'll weigh myself from time to time, and hopefully I'll get to 98 pounds, which is my goal, but if it takes forever, as long as I feel good and I'm continuing to develop lean muscle, I am happy.

So happy.

🎵 PLAYLIST HIGHLIGHTS

My Long Run Mix

I've added new and old favorites.

Corner of the Sky – From the *Pippin* New Broadway Cast Recording, featuring the dreamy Matthew James Thomas

To Be Surprised – Sondre Lerche

Latch – Disclosure

Go Do – Jonsi

Could You Be Loved – Bob Marley

Got 2 Luv U – Sean Paul

Timebomb – Kylie Minogue

The Bitch of Living – From *Spring Awakening*

You've Been a Friend to Me – Bryan Adams

I'll Stand By You – Pretenders

Dog Days Are Over – Florence + the Machine

Liquid Lunch – Caro Emerald

Saturday in the Park – Chicago

Time after Time – Cyndi Lauper

Kingston Town – UB40

Don't Matter – Akon

Electric Avenue – Eddy Grant

SexyBack – Justin Timberlake

Summer – Calvin Harris

Funkytown – Lipps

The Safety Dance – Men Without Hats

While My Guitar Gently Weeps – George Harrison

Lakehouse – Of Monsters and Men

Home – Edward Sharpe & the Magnetic Zeros

Rhythm of Love – Plain White Ts

Happy – Pharrell Williams

CHAPTER 6 – REUEL

Everyone gets to that point where they're thinking, *I've been working so hard—I should be done.*

So one thing I knew I would be doing consistently with Carolee was repeatedly going over what needed to be done and discussing the same things over and over.

She kept asking me why, and I kept telling her achieving results is not easy.

When you don't have background knowledge and you don't have the experience of working out consistently to your limits, it's hard to take what someone else says seriously unless you're seeing results.

Carolee would ask me, "Why don't I feel it in this spot?"

"Why am I not making the gains I thought I'd be making by now?"

When I think about my experience with Carolee, I remember that feeling of euphoria I had when she held a side plank in correct form for 30 seconds. It took weeks—maybe two months—before she went from 15 to 30 seconds executing it perfectly. I thought, *finally she's ready to be pushed.*

As an experiment, I asked her to hold a wall sit for five minutes. I had no idea whether she could do this.

She sat on that wall for five minutes! I was surprised at how dedicated Carolee was.

I saw she was serious, and I thought, *Now we're cookin'!*

There were some things we didn't do because we hadn't built the foundation to perform them correctly or because they caused her pain. Carolee and I talked a lot about the difference between pain and burning, and because she was so new at this, I was extremely cautious. I'd ask her— to her great annoyance at times—how are you feeling? Is it pain or burning? Usually, if I wasn't convinced she knew the difference, I'd say, "Give me two more, great job, take a break."

One thing I wanted to do with Carolee was evaluate frequently to see if she could execute exercises correctly. As we approached super high reps of exercises—even up to 50 reps—I'd say, "That's it, we can't do this anymore." To make progress we'd modify or switch to a different exercise.

As a trainer, I can't have someone doing 50 reps.

Early on, the arm bike was Carolee's go-to cardio machine. This was my idea, because I thought this would help her burn calories but more importantly help her feel as though we were doing exactly what she wanted, since she often focused on her arms.

I knew she could benefit from running on the treadmill, especially if I could get her to do interval runs—but I thought, *let's keep building her confidence first*. Gradually I began sneaking a few minutes with her on the treadmill into our sessions.

Everyone's different, so it's hard to gauge how someone is going to react to your comments and suggestions. I know Carolee had a hard time getting comfortable with the idea of someone (me) watching her so closely. At first, I wanted her to perform exercises in front of a mirror, so she could pay attention to her form, but she was too uncomfortable looking at herself, so I put that idea aside.

There were two pivotal points that stood out for me when I thought back about Carolee's training. The first was I knew she was dedicated when she started to come in early to run before our 6:00 a.m. sessions, as well as when we didn't even have a session. The second time was when she started using the mirrors.

Good for you, I thought.

CHAPTER 7 – FITNESS IS EVERYTHING

Day 285, January 8, 2015

> *"Potentially lovely, perpetually human."*
> —Regina Spektor, "Open"

So much about being disciplined has to do with momentum. It's just easier to show up and go full-out when you're in your groove.

When you've got the flu, or when it's that time of the month when you want to be in bed with a heating pad (yeah, I know—forever young), that's when keeping your focus becomes especially challenging.

You've got to listen to your body, because if you push, you're setting yourself up for injury. But if you take off time, it's hard to get back in it.

Practicing social distancing, where possible, aside, all of us have to go to work, school, and honor commitments when we're not feeling 100 percent well. When Mia was little, she performed with a children's choir when she wasn't feeling great at an event honoring Audrey Hepburn. On the way home, I caught her eye in the rearview mirror.

"I need to find someone who can teach me how to sing with a cold," she sighed.

What I noticed most about running on Sunday while I was sick enough to go out and buy boxes of tissues was how depleted I felt. By mile 8, I hit a wall and had to stop because I was lightheaded. I turned off my MapMyRun app so I wouldn't be tempted to start running again, and I walked the three miles back to Bethesda. It was a scary feeling, especially since the only other times I've experienced it were at the gym around a ton of people certified to perform CPR.

I had been doing low-key workouts all week and hadn't been in the pool.

Mentally I was irritable, so by Sunday, I needed to get out and run. I opted not to run with the MCRRC, which was doing an 11-mile run out and back on the Capital Crescent Trail, because it was pouring rain early on Sunday. When the weather cleared up, I planned to do the same run as the club, and for the first five or six miles I was in my zone. The weather was moist and warm, and I was outlining a writing assignment in my head. I felt great.

By the time I reached Fletcher's Cove, I should have realized I had become dehydrated, because I did not need to use the restroom. I ran another half mile beyond Fletcher's before turning back. The drinking fountain at Fletcher's was out of order, and I hadn't brought a water bottle with me because the previous Sunday I had done my run with it attached to a belt around my waist and never used it.

When I finally stopped at mile 8, I was at the DC-MD line, where there is a working water fountain. I drank a little and started walking back.

I've been thinking about hydration as well as fuel during workouts and runs for some time now and probably talk about it obsessively with anyone who'll listen. I'm convinced I need to find a way to hydrate without worrying about finding a pit stop. I also felt my gait was off with the water hanging around my waist. I'm planning to try a handheld contraption this weekend, but I might need to learn how to run with a water belt. Plenty of people do it.

It's tricky, because I don't think many of us appreciate how much water our bodies need and why. Or maybe it's only me who doesn't get it.

The way Lord Baltimore explained it, we are mostly water by far. We're designed to regulate our hydration status carefully through (1) the brain and the thirst response and (2) the kidneys. When the kidneys filter the blood, they can hold on to more or less water depending on the body's needs.

The body regulates both fluid status and temperature. It controls temperature mostly by regulating perspiration.

So when you're running or exercising vigorously and perspiring, you can potentially become dehydrated.

In the situation where the body has to choose what's more important, a. bringing the temperature down by perspiring more or b. maintaining good hydration of tissues by reducing perspiration, it will choose the latter. Essentially your body will allow your temperature to rise to dangerously high levels in order to preserve fluid balance to maintain blood pressure.

The purpose of maintaining blood pressure is to get oxygen and nutrients—including water—to the tissues, especially the brain.

The link here for me is that when I become dehydrated, the first symptom after thirst is weakness and feeling faint, even to the point of passing out.

For months, my internist has been monitoring my high blood pressure, which may be related to my physical activity. Since Sunday, Lord Baltimore has made a point to check it. It's been all over the place, and it was especially high on Monday night after I smashed my new car into a pole pulling out of a parking space after getting an emergency bikini wax.

It came down after I had a shot of Bushmills.

I'm certain I hit the pole because I wasn't functioning at 100 percent, so I'm not sure why I thought I could exercise as if I was at the top of my game.

All I want to eat is hot and sour soup from the local Chinese carry out.

On Tuesday, when I was teleworking during the snowstorm that hit Washington early in the morning, I went to take one of my granola bars from the footed glass cookie jar on my kitchen counter, and the lid slipped out of my hand and smashed into a million pieces.

I've had that jar on my counter for as long as I can remember, and I was horrified at the violence of it all.

I'm finally on the other side of this, but I promise to go slow this weekend. I could barely get to three miles on the treadmill this morning, and the only reason why I was able to keep going from two to three was because the person on the treadmill next to me was up for having a conversation.

🎵 PLAYLIST HIGHLIGHTS

I've been back to listening to my Turkey Chase Mix, with a little bit of Nashville thrown in.

1234 – Feist

Club Can't Handle Me – Flo Rida

Ooh La La – Goldfrapp

Coastin' – Zion I & K. Flay

Down with the Trumpets – Rizzle Kicks

Timber – Pitbull

Comme un Enfant – Yelle

Crazy Kids – Kesha

I Am the Best – 2NET1

Sabali – Amadou & Mariam

Come with Me Now – Kongos

We Are One – Pitbull

212 – Azealia Banks

Tainted Love – Soft Cell

In da Club – 50 Cent

We Run the Night – Havana Brown

Pieces of the People We Love – The Rapture

We Sink – Chvrches

Lovers' Eyes – Mumford and Sons

Mozart's House – Clean Bandit

A Little Bit of Me – Melissa Etheridge

Take Me to Church – Hozier

Carry On – Fun.

Come Over – Clean Bandit

Faded – Zhu

Rhythm of Love – Plain White Ts

Run-Around – Blues Traveler

Ripple – Grateful Dead

Latch – Disclosure

Lakehouse – Of Monsters and Men

Need You Now – Antebellum

Boys 'Round Here – Blake Shelton

Rewind – Rascal Flatts

Day 293, January 16, 2015

> *"I came in like a wrecking ball."*
> —Kar Play, "Wrecking Ball"
> (House piano extended version)

I'm not sure if Really Smart was trying to distract me as she was digging into my right glute when she started to engage me in a conversation about the different kinds of muscle fibers.

"You know the difference between fast and slow twitch muscle fibers, right?" she asked. I'm flattered when Really Smart thinks I have any knowledge here.

"No."

Slow twitch muscle fibers are endurance muscles, so for running these are great, and they're the ones you want to develop, she said. They use oxygen efficiently and fire more slowly, so they take more time to fatigue.

We never got to fast twitch muscle fibers, so I think I can leave them aside for a while.

The subject came up because I'm continuing to do long runs on Sundays—I'm scheduled to do 12 miles this Sunday with the MCRRC—but I'm experiencing significant muscle fatigue around eight miles and major glute burn for days. Really Smart wants me to rethink my "exercise prescription" (seriously) now that I'm doing long-distance running.

So far, my goals have focused on calorie burn and toning and strengthening the muscles in my core so I can exercise without injury. Now she wants to take a look at how I'm strengthening my slow twitch muscle fibers in order to increase my muscle endurance, which is how a muscle performs over time.

For this, she introduced me to the overload principle, which according to the articles she gave me to read while she stuck me with a million dry needles simply means that if you want to improve muscle performance, you need to add load that exceeds the metabolic capacity of the muscle.

So how does this relate to me and increasing my muscle endurance by developing my slow twitch muscle fibers? For endurance training, Really Smart said the idea is to increase the time a muscle contraction is sustained or the number of reps performed, as opposed to progressively increasing resistance (or load).

Although strength training (adding load) is also one of my 2015 goals, for now I need to find the right level of resistance that exceeds the metabolic capacity of the muscle, but at the same time increase the number of reps to build endurance so I will be able to run beyond eight miles without discomfort.

I don't think it's a one-or-the-other approach to training, but it might be. I haven't had a conversation with Buff about this, as we're still getting comfortable working together. And I'm just coming back to the land of the living after having the flu. Really Smart's handout also discussed the "specificity of training" and whether my time would be better spent actually running—particularly running hills—rather than training in the gym. I talked to Really Smart about this, but because of the glute burn, she said, no, not yet. While she has told me in the past that the only way to train to run long-distance is to run long distance, for the moment, I need to give my sorry glutes a rest. With this in mind, I'm doing one long run per week and only one to two miles on the treadmill before any training or other gym workouts when I'm not in the pool.

We also talked (again) about muscular rest and recovery, and I need to be way more strategic about this. She reminded me that there are different kinds of muscle fatigue. The most obvious is the temporary state of exhaustion (failure) that leads to a decrease in muscle strength. I need to be tuned in to when to stop in order to allow sufficient time for the fatigued muscle to rest and recover.

This isn't so easy, especially when I'm running, and I have a feeling I'm not letting my muscles recover sufficiently. I know I need help with this. I'm working on it and hope I'll get it right, because I enjoy the long runs and want to be able to do them without fatigue or the pain that comes with muscle fatigue.

***

My workout friend Robyn Shields shared her fantastic vegetarian split pea recipe, which I'm including here because I don't want you to go another day without the perfect soup recipe. It's easy and elegant served with a dollop of crème fraiche.

ROBYN'S VEGETARIAN SPLIT PEA SOUP

Serves 6–8

Ingredients

2.5 cups dried split peas (1 pound), rinsed and picked over

10 cups vegetable stock

2 tsp. olive oil

1 large onion, diced

1 clove garlic, minced

2 cups sliced carrots

2 cups sliced celery

2 bay leaves

1 Tbsp. dried oregano

1 large bunch parsley, chopped

Salt and pepper to taste

Juice of 1 lemon

Croutons or crème fraiche (optional, as garnish)

Instructions

1. Heat olive oil in a soup pot over medium heat.

2. When it's hot, add the onions and sauté for a few minutes until they soften and begin to sweat. Add the garlic and sauté for another minute.

3. Add the carrots, celery, peas, stock, and herbs to the pot and bring to a boil.

4. Reduce to a simmer, and, stirring occasionally, let the soup go for 2 hours, partially covered.

5. Add the lemon juice and salt and pepper to taste.

6. Allow the soup to simmer for another few minutes, then remove the bay leaves.

I use an immersion blender to puree the soup; Robyn throws the whole thing into the Vitamix, so either will work. If you use the Vitamix, you can probably cook the soup around 90 minutes. If you're using the immersion blender, you'll need the full 2 hours to completely dissolve the peas.

***

🎵 PLAYLIST HIGHLIGHTS

The other night at dinner I had the pleasure of sitting next to Palmer Hefferan, the hipster sound designer of *Cherokee,* which opened at the Woolly Mammoth Theater Company on February 9. You know I asked her what she's listening to. I'm not a huge Miley Cyrus fan, but I love the Kar Play house remix of "Wrecking Ball" that she turned me on to, as well as Sia's epic "Chandelier." I forgot how transcendental house music can be. Here are some of my favorites (and a few other non-house additions).

Mozart's House – Clean Bandit (featuring Love Ssega)

Wrecking Ball (House piano extended instrumental)
– Kar Play

Don't You Worry Child (featuring John Martin) –
Swedish House Mafia

Save the World (Zedd remix) – Swedish House Mafia

#Selfie – The Chainsmokers

Every Teardrop Is a Waterfall – Coldplay vs. Swedish
House Mafia (live)

Gucci Mane – Trap House 3

House Party – Meek Mill

Chandelier – Sia

Bluebird Wine – Emmylou Harris & Rodney Crowell

Day 310, February 2, 2015

"Prepared to be surprised."
—Sondre Lerche, "To Be Surprised"

Whoever said the great thing about running is all you have
to do is lace up your sneakers and go was not introduced to
the concept of *gear*.

Here's what I've got on me to do a run in 17-degree weather:

◊ Under Armour Women's UA Storm Heather T-Neck (Absolute genius.)

◊ Under Armour ColdGear Fitted Long Sleeve Crew

◊ Under Armour ColdGear ankle running pants or Lululemon lined ankle running pants (I love Lululemon pants, but they are expensive. UA is a little more slippery, but the ColdGear is fantastic— I just bought these in purple.)

◊ Under Armour cap—Amazon has them in packs of five (They get soaking wet, so you have to wash them after a run).

◊ face mask

◊ North Face ETIP running gloves

◊ iPhone armband

◊ iPhone with MapMyFitness app (Audio coaching turned ON.)

◊ Urbanears earbuds

◊ hand warmers

◊ water belt

◊ Voltaren Gel (For my glutes and hamstrings before a run.)

- ◊ Swedish Fish/gummy bears

- ◊ trail mix

- ◊ Smartwool ultralight socks or Balegas

- ◊ custom inserts from Road Runner Sports (Like orthotics but cheaper.)

- ◊ Brooks Adrenaline ASR 11 GTX Trail-Running Shoes with a Gore-Tex membrane (Great in cold or wet weather.)

I realize I'm like a broken record here, but you have to be strategic about your fitness if you want to see results. I was enjoying doing weekly long runs with the MCRRC (e.g., 13.02 miles on Sunday from Grosvenor to the National Zoo in the pouring rain), but it was taking days for my glutes to recover, preventing me from running during the week, so I wondered whether that was making any sense.

Although I was getting an awesome calorie burn on the long runs (982), I wasn't getting anything close to that on the elliptical or in the pool during the week. I talked to Really Smart about this, and she told me to back off from the long runs and stick to mileage below my pain threshold, at least for a while.

I'm worried about this because I'm registered to run in the D.C. Rock 'n' Roll Half Marathon on March 14, but I don't think I have a choice.

Last weekend while I was at Vassar, I ran three miles on the treadmill and did some core work on the mat. Back at the gym during the week, I was able to run four miles on the treadmill and cross-train in the pool and on the recumbent bike and the elliptical. This past Saturday, I did my favorite eight-mile run from Bethesda to Georgetown on the Capital Crescent Trail in my new UA Storm gear and felt absolutely great (and stylish). So, while I miss running with the club and the amazing rush I was getting by going more than 10 miles, I have zero glute pain today.

Clutch.

***

Last week, when the weather in Washington was beyond miserable, I was talking with my friend Robyn Shields in the Equinox locker room while we were getting ready for work after our six o'clock morning workout. We agreed how incredibly hard it is to get out of bed and to the gym in the mornings these days. It's tough after work, too.

These are real challenges, and visualizing results is what gets me out the door six days a week.

It's helpful to get my gear ready before I go to sleep, but it's even more important now since it is so cold in the mornings. I need to get my gym stuff on super quick and race to the kitchen to make a cup of coffee before I am tempted to crawl back under the covers. I know I'm addicted to exercise, but I'm also human and have the same desire as everyone else to skip the morning drive to the gym.

Robyn and I talked about how much we have to push ourselves. For me, and I suspect for Robyn too, everything comes together when you keep your fitness goals on the front burner. I talked recently with Adorable about my foot pain after eight miles, and he reminded me how important it is for me to work on balance, which I had forgotten about or completely ignored. Running is essentially like balancing on one foot, since both of your feet are never on the ground at the same time.

I feel like it's a waste to work on balance while I'm at the gym, but I think there's a payoff that's as epic as the definition you get in your arms when you work with weights or do push-ups.

Like running long distances without pain.

I'll do whatever I need to get to that place. Cross-training, gear, balance exercises, I'm not snubbing any of it. And working with a new trainer takes effort, too. Buff is highly skilled, but he's changing things up.

When Buff started to incorporate more (and heavier) weights, you know I checked in with Adorable.

"I think it's a good idea to bring more weight into the mix," Adorable said.

So okay, I'm going with it. We're adding more load, and when we're not doing that, we're adding more reps. Buff is starting to get me, and although he's tough, he's also sweet.

The bottom line is, I'm making progress and seeing results.

***

Just one thing about last night's Super Bowl. Even if you're a Seahawks fan, you've gotta give rookie Malcolm Butler major kudos for his amazing goal-line interception in the last seconds of the game. Wow, talk about focus. That guy's got it.

🎵 PLAYLIST HIGHLIGHTS

Can't wait for the Grammys next Sunday so I can fill in what I missed in 2014.

My Evolving Long Run Mix:

Bluebird Wine – Emmylou Harris and Rodney Crowell

Wrecking Ball (House piano extended version) – Kar Play

To Be Surprised – Sondre Lerche

Go Do – Jonsi

Latch featuring Sam Smith – Disclosure

Take Me to Church – Hozier

We Run the Night – Pitbull

Me and My Broken Heart – Rixton

Don't Tell 'Em – Jeremih

Every Teardrop Is a Waterfall – Coldplay Until Now Deluxe Version

Faded – Shu

Sabali – Amadou and Mariam

Corner of the Sky – Matthew James Thomas

Could You Be Loved – Bob Marley

Timebomb – Kylie Minogue

Got 2 Luv U – Sean Paul

I'll Stand By You – Pretenders

I Will Wait – Mumford and Sons

Dog Days Are Over – Florence + the Machine

The Con – Tegan and Sara

Closer to the Sun – Slightly Stoopid

Liquid Lunch – Caro Emerald

Kingston Town – UB40

Don't Matter – Akon

Electric Avenue extended version – Eddy Grant

SexyBack – Justin Timberlake

Right Round – Flo Rida

The Safety Dance – Men Without Hats

Run-Around – Blues Traveler

Come Over – Clean Bandit

Lakehouse – Of Monsters and Men

212 – Azealia Banks

Tainted Love – Soft Cell

We Are One (Ole Ole) – Pitbull

Comme Un Enfant – Yelle

Come With Me Now – Kongos

Paper Planes – M.I.A.

Day 321, February 13, 2015

> *"Boom, boom, boom."*
> —Katy Perry, "Firework"

It's a bonanza morning when you wake up and nothing hurts. It's even better when you have some soreness—the good kind—because that's what you want. No pain, no stiffness, no numbness.

That only lasts for a day, and then you're back to figuring out what you did to cause a strain in your left glute just when your right glute is absolutely A-OK.

This came up earlier in the week, because just as both glutes were being very quiet, I was having some significant pain on the top of my left shoulder, which was inhibiting my mobility and preventing me from doing any kind of challenging planks. After I told Buff I was too uncomfortable to push through, he handed me a five-pound weight and showed me how to use my hips to create momentum that would allow my arm to swing like a pendulum.

"Try to incorporate this into your warm-up to loosen up the shoulder muscles," he said

"Okay, so add this to rolling, arm swings, walking on the treadmill, using the recumbent bike, leg lifts with ankle weights, balancing on one leg, stretching..."

"And repeat," quipped a trainer on the mat, rolling his IT band.

Buff was trying to put all of this into perspective by telling me I am working very hard, so I should expect to take extra time for muscle recovery.

"On those days when you need to let your muscles repair themselves, do light stretching and walking," he said.

I've heard this advice before from Really Smart, Adorable, and Triathlete, but it seems counterintuitive, and I haven't found a way to get myself to take time off beyond one day per week. Part of the problem is I don't want to take time off, so I keep thinking I will toughen up. I'm in much better shape than I was even two months ago, but on some days I can't carry the laundry basket upstairs.

***

I wish I could let my hair grow so I can pull it back into a pony tail when I run—you know, the kind that sticks out of a baseball cap. So cute. But I can't get past the stage where my hair is soaking wet at the back of my neck. It doesn't help when my Dessange Paris hairstylist works out at Equinox Bethesda and gives me the evil eye when he sees me after I've run on the treadmill. He usually wins, and before you know it, I've got the latest short cut, which I'll admit is so practical and comfortable.

***

I told my team at work I would be leaving for a detail assignment in Kingston.

"How will you train for your half marathon?"

"I'm so glad you asked me that question," I said.

If I'm a little too out there on the personal stuff, I'd say that train has left the station.

I told them I plan to run in the mornings before I head to the embassy and figure I won't have too many distractions because I'll be working long hours. I'll use my weekends to travel to Jamaica's gorgeous beaches and swim in the Caribbean and should be in great shape when I return to Washington a day before the race.

Hey, I'm a team player.

♪ PLAYLIST HIGHLIGHTS

Here's where I'm at with getting ready for the Rock 'n' Roll Half Marathon with my rock 'n' roll mix. Wherever possible I'm listening to the live versions of songs, especially rock songs, because the party atmosphere and cheering crowds energize me. My running group is doing 14 miles on Saturday instead of Sunday this weekend because of the weather. I'm planning to do this run, and it'll be my last long run until the race.

Take It Easy (live) – Eagles

Sunshine of Your Love – Cream

Livin' on a Prayer (live) – Bon Jovi

Born to Be Wild (live) – Steppenwolf

Aqualung (live) – Jethro Tull

Ramblin' Man – Allman Bros

Don't Stop Believin' – Journey

Nights in White Satin – Moody Blues

Can't Get It Out of My Head – Electric Light Orchestra

I'm Your Captain/Closer to Home – Grand Funk Railroad

Take Me to the River (live) – Talking Heads

Give a Little Bit (live) – Goo Dolls

In the Air Tonight (live) – Phil Collins – so great

Go Your Own Way (live) – Fleetwood Mac

Firework – Katy Perry

Welcome to New York – Taylor Swift (Mia added this.)

I'll Stand By You – Pretenders

Could You Be Loved – Bob Marley

While My Guitar Gently Weeps – George Harrison

Truckin' – Grateful Dead

Bohemian Rhapsody – Queen

American Idiot – Green Day

Moondance – Van Morrison

Closing Time – Semisonic

Semi-Charmed Life – Third Eye Blind

Heaven – Los Lonely Boys

Knockin' on Heaven's Door – Guns and Roses

Satellite – Guster

Somebody to Love – Jefferson Airplane

How to Save a Life – The Fray

Brandy – Looking Glass

Because the Night – Patti Smith

Sympathy for the Devil – Rolling Stones

Bad Day – Daniel Powter

Drunken Lullabies – Flogging Molly

Dream On (live) – Aerosmith

Day 327, February 19, 2015

> *"All it takes is just a simple oh-oh-oh."*
> —Clean Bandit, "Come Over"

Enter supplements. As in whey powder and casein powder.

My long run on Saturday at Lake Needwood in Rockville—16 miles total; 14 running and two walking—was as hard as it gets. This was my first long run since January 18 and my last before the D.C. Rock 'n' Roll Half Marathon on March 14.

I know some of it was my own fault. Like an idiot, I did not bring water, but hear me out. I was running with the MCRRC, and we were doing a 14-mile in and out run with a water break at mile 7. The only information I had about a bathroom break was at the trail head, so I figured I'd tank up two hours before the run, get water at 7, and run back.

My pace group decided to do 12 miles instead of 14. I opted to keep going because I didn't have any water with me, and two other runners decided to join me. But here's what happened. The water break was actually at mile 8, and there were bathrooms. I know it sounds crazy, but going that extra mile without hydration depleted me, and my muscles were starting to hurt.

I tried to drink a good amount, but I know now from experience it was too little, too late. I also had a handful of trail mix and Swedish Fish, but nothing helped.

I drank some chocolate milk in the car, and as soon as I got home, I googled "Why am I so sore after a long run?"

Articles on protein supplements were practically screaming at me. I've been gradually adding more protein into my diet, especially after runs and workouts, but what I'm learning is that whey powder, unlike eggs for example, digests lightning fast. The rapid delivery of amino acids to your muscle cells helps you fast-track repairing your shredded tissues before they start swelling and causing the kind of pain that prevents you from exercising.

The articles recommended having a whey powder shake before and after long runs and swimming about 2,000 yards within 12 hours or so. Luckily, I had whey in the fridge because Adin, as a dancer, had been taking it for years, and I swam Sunday morning.

I talked with Buff about this Monday morning and then with Really Smart later in the day during our session. Both gave me that "I can't believe you didn't know this" look that I've seen more often than I like.

But as Really Smart pointed out, you have to be careful with protein supplements because (1) they can be caloric and (2) you can bulk up, and if you're working on developing lean muscle this can be a problem. That's where casein protein comes in. It digests more slowly, and apparently many runners take it at bedtime.

So I'm adding these two to my regimen but being hyper-cognizant of how they're making me feel, so far so good, especially first thing in the morning before I head to the gym. I'm mixing almost a full scoop with 6 ounces of freshly squeezed orange juice, which makes the most delicious creamsicle concoction that takes me back to my childhood summers on Long Island.

***

So here's another interesting challenge. I have just boarded my connecting flight to Kingston, Jamaica, where I'll be working for the next three weeks.

No family support, no Buff, no Really Smart, no Adorable. I was talking to Adin on the phone during the car ride to the airport this morning, and we were going through a checklist to figure out what I forgot. We got to my workout clothes, which by the way have their own suitcase (I'm not a light packer), and he asked me if I had my physical therapy gear. My weights, bands, and so on.

"No, I didn't pack those."

"Was there a reason you decided not to pack them or is that what you forgot?"

"I just figured taking them was over the top, and I'll see what the fitness center has at my hotel."

I've got so much on my plate the next few weeks. So much stuff to learn for work and so much training to do on my own. I'll let you know how it goes.

P.S. I forgot my hairbrush.

Day 337, March 1, 2015

> *"Sing with me just for today."*
> —Aerosmith, "Dream On"

"Fitness is everything."

Meet Rasta Dave, my guide this morning during a seven-mile hike on Strawberry Hill in the Jamaican Blue Mountains. He's not really *my* guide. The guy is legendary and practically has celebrity status any place you go in Kingston.

The whole thing took about three hours, and it was serious hiking, all of it either flat or downhill. At the bottom, in Gordon Town, we took a taxi back up the mountain.

The path was rocky and steep, and I'm so glad I did not wear my favorite blue Brooks, which would have been destroyed. I only decided to change into my low Frye boots at the last minute as I was waiting in the hotel lobby for my ride. I looked online and saw the TripAdvisor comments about the terrain. I'm glad I had hard-sole shoes with me.

Dave was pleasant, and our conversation flowed. The air was completely still, and for quite a while we did not hear a single sound. After I commented how absolutely quiet it was, we talked about the flowering trees and bushes all around us. I thought I spotted the national flower of Jamaica, but when I pointed it out, neither one of us could remember the name, but he was sure we were looking at what he called a garlic flower.

He told me Jamaicans work hard from Monday to Friday and party hard on Friday and Saturday nights. They're inside on Saturday mornings. Kids are doing their homework. That's why it's so quiet right now, he said.

The topic of fitness came up after we passed by avocado, banana, and plantain trees, and then bushes with pineapples and trees with mangos, mandarins, and breadfruit. He broke open a cacao bean for me and showed me what ackee, the national fruit of Jamaica, looks like. We were in coffee country so there were coffee bushes everywhere. It reminded me of Napa's wine country, where you pass one grapevine after another.

Dave talked about how essential fruit is to the Jamaican diet and how much he values eating healthfully and being fit. He told me about the potato pudding he makes in a coal pot, and how easy and plentiful it is for Jamaicans to take what they need from the trees all along the roads.

Soon things started to get busy up on the mountain. At a certain point, the road ends, and the only way for people to get things to their homes or businesses is to leave their cars and carry their goods on their heads. We passed men carrying cartons of glass beverages. We crossed four footbridges over the river, and we said hello to a woman washing clothes in the river just before one of several falls. Dave spent a few minutes catching up with a young woman hiking up the mountain as she was plugged in to her iPod. She told Dave she's training to join the Jamaican army.

"That's the way to get a good job," Dave commented to me.

He guides up to three hikes a day, and he has been doing this for years. He has two daughters in Boston, one a physician, and he loves it when they visit him in Jamaica. He has no desire to live in Boston, where right now it's bitter cold.

As our conversation meandered, Dave tried to provide me with context for the popular music in Kingston, especially for reggae dancehall music, which has essentially replaced reggae here. Dave said most people in Kingston consider reggae old-fashioned.

He likes Chronixx, the dancehall artist who's got a "message," which is what reggae, Bob Marley's reggae, is about. Most of dancehall is about an electronic sound/beat, so Dave isn't the biggest fan. I feel the same way, but I'm warming to it. He told me Bob Marley's manager had discovered Chronixx, so that gave the young artist some street cred.

Toward the end we were both quiet. The altitude was making me lightheaded. The taxi headed back up the mountain switchbacks with ease, and the radio station played dancehall intermingled with classic reggae.

As I gazed out the window from the back seat, I thought how much I agree with Dave.

Fitness and health are everything.

***

The thing about traveling for work is that I'm never a tourist. I can do exploring on the weekends, but I'm always aware that I'm there to do my job.

It also means I am by myself during many of the off hours, and as an extrovert, I'm spending a lot of time talking with hotel staff, my driver, and other business travelers having dinner at one of the hotel bars.

I'm not opposed to driving myself around Kingston, but the cars are on the other side of the road, and there isn't enough time for me to become confident I wouldn't crash into someone head on.

So I have Nigel, my driver. He's also a great ambassador of Kingston and astoundingly chatty for a guy, especially at six thirty in the morning.

From the outset, Nigel has taken me under his wing and provided Kingston 101.

"Drivers can be aggressive in Kingston," Nigel told me. "It's totally different in the rural areas, in the country."

There's no *soon come* here.

"Ocho Rios? Montego Bay? Port Antonio?"

"Yeah man. In the country it's different."

Nigel set me straight that in Kingston they say, "yeah man," meaning "that's right," while in the country, they say, "yah mon" or "yah man."

"We have a different patois here," he said.

This morning when he dropped me off at the top of Strawberry Hill, he spent the 45-minute drive talking to me about the Kingston vibe, the abundance of agriculture, and the family culture. He's got a daughter who lives in the United Kingdom with her Jamaican mother, and friends everywhere.

By the way, Dave was Nigel's idea. He practically planned my day for me—the hike, lunch, pedicure (okay, that was my two cents). Afterward, when he picked me up, I told him about my lunch at Strawberry Hill and mentioned that although it's high season for tourists right now, the place seemed empty.

"It has cottages scattered about and everything is private. Celebrities and writers come up there for privacy. The place is full—you just won't ever see anybody there. That's why people like it."

Okay then.

***

For what it's worth, I've always thought life was good in Jamaica. Sure, a lot of people are really, really poor, and the country has a high violent crime rate. But that's not the point. The many Jamaicans I come in contact with every day are personable and genuinely nice.

This is of course at odds with the fact that Jamaican law prohibits certain sexual activities and is often used to target LGBT individuals. There is also an "antibuggery" law that prohibits consensual same-sex sexual conduct between men.

Negative attitudes toward LGBT issues are widespread in Jamaican pop culture and politics. Often Jamaicans say the church opposes homosexuality. And there are a lot of churches in Jamaica. Especially because of Bob Marley's "one love" message, the pop culture thing perplexes me.

Last week Secretary of State Kerry appointed career Foreign Service Officer Randy Berry as the special envoy on LGBT issues. I suspect he'll be visiting Jamaica.

I'm diggin' that.

🎵 PLAYLIST HIGHLIGHTS

I'm listening to reggae dancehall, but I'm also getting comfortable with my rock 'n' roll mix to prepare for my race on March 14. Here are a few of my favorites right now.

Don't Stop Believin' – Journey

Tiny Dancer (Live) – Elton John (Patrick Gatti, who was in Kingston on business from Florida, highly encouraged me to add this one.)

Dream On – Aerosmith

Go Your Own Way – Fleetwood Mac

Bohemian Rhapsody – Queen

Beat It – Michael Jackson

Getting Married – Yellow Man

It's Magic – Dennis Brown

Here Comes Trouble – Chronixx

Smile Jamaica – Chronixx

Too Rude – Half Pint

Day 342, March 6, 2015

"If we show up, we gon' show out."
—Mark Ronson, "Uptown Funk"

Now that I've been in Kingston for nearly three weeks, I'm settling into a fitness routine just as I'm getting ready to head back to Washington for my first half marathon.

My challenges:

◊ The hotel fitness center tries hard but misses, at least for me. There are two functional treadmills, about six upright bikes, one weight machine I recognize, a few mats, and a couple of benches. No elliptical (it's broken), no recumbent bikes, no Bosu ball, no rollers.

◊ Since I get picked up early, I'm not able to exercise before work, which is my usual routine.

◊ Because I am learning something new that requires critical thinking, I am hungry all day and eating more food than usual.

◊ And eating all meals out.

◊ No trainer.

◊ On the plus side: It's still daylight when I return to the hotel after work, so I can walk or run in Emancipation Park across from my hotel. There's a (cushioned) jogging path that loops around the park. Each lap is about .33 mile and has a nice little incline for half a lap. It's funny being on the path with runners/walkers who pass on the right just like the cars.

◊ After doing a three-mile run or walk, I try to head to the fitness center to do core work (focusing on my back and my abs) and my PT exercises on my legs and glutes.

◊ Two times per week I've been able to do 45 minutes in the hotel pool. It's not a good idea to do this on Tuesdays, which is barbeque night poolside, I learned. All was well last week until hotel staff started to use skimmers to clean the pool to get ready for the party while I was still in there.

◊ The Marines run a boot camp at the Embassy. Think spidermen, leap frogs, burpees, backward crab walking, all on the concrete. I'm glad I did it once.

◊ Okay, sorry, I have to say it: the weather is simply warm and perfect. This was my first experience running in warm weather since I just started running in the fall. There are definitely challenges, but my muscles warm up much more quickly than in 7 degrees, so that's good.

Since I tweaked my left gluteus medius sidestepping during the 5.5k Sagicor race the first weekend I was here, I did not run for seven days. I know now I could have used the stairs in the embassy or in the hotel to get in some cardio, so I will try to add that into the mix this week if I need to.

I'm aware my lack of cardio will definitely be a factor on race day, but at this point I can only do what I can do. I've had support from Adorable and Buff while I'm here, and both have offered great suggestions for how to make my workouts pay off during my run.

Late Sunday I received an email from my running club coach with tips for preparing for a half marathon. One tip I love is visualizing the race as two 6-mile races. Genius. Another is to run relaxed, easy pace three-milers a few times during the week or two preceding the race.

I tried my first three-miler outside since the Sagicor race last night, and it went fine. I'm sore today, but it's a good sore (so far), so my plan is to do another run early Saturday morning before taking a day trip to the beach and doing laps in the pool on Sunday.

I'm trying to prepare mentally more than anything else, because there's little I can do at this point to prepare physically except maybe injure myself.

At least I'm not craving sugar. I've been having protein at every meal: eggs and callaloo and whole wheat toast for breakfast, salad or vegetables with jerk chicken for lunch (most days) at the embassy, and fish for dinner at the hotel. In between meals I'm having pineapple and papaya and any kind of nuts I can find. Almonds are too expensive in Jamaica, so they aren't readily available.

My favorite item on the menu for dinner—other than on barbeque night or Italian night—is the blackened red snapper sandwich with fries. Except the bartenders and waiters at the hotel know to hold all the starch from my plate—no bread, no fries. Instead, they just serve the blackened red snapper with steamed vegetables and lettuce and tomato. Perfect.

***

I'm not planning to take this approach during my race on March 14, but I've been thinking a lot about Jen Miller's NYT article "Real Runners Do Take Walk Breaks." Miller, a long-distance runner, runs for 9 minutes, walks for 1 minute, and then repeats.

She refers to a study in the *Journal of Science and Medicine in Sport* that showed runners who took regular walking breaks during a race had the same finish time as when they had run the entire race.

In addition, runners who took walking breaks had less muscle pain after the race.

Miller says running coach and Olympic runner Jeff Galloway pioneered the walk/run approach to racing. It's worth reading about him.

I typically try not to walk when I'm running—except maybe on a steep hill—because I find my muscles tighten up, which makes it difficult to resume running. I notice this when I take a water or bathroom break and try to do a few stretches before I get back out onto the trail.

Especially because of the discomfort I experience after running long distances, the run/walk approach might make perfect sense for me.

🎵 PLAYLIST HIGHLIGHTS

Uptown Funk – Mark Ronson featuring Bruno Mars

Happy – Pharrell Williams

Sk8er Boi – Avril Lavigne

Firework – Katy Perry

Walk Away – Jasmine V

Welcome to New York – Taylor Swift

Time of Our Lives – Pitbull

Don't Tell 'Em – Jeremih

Me and My Broken Heart – Rixton

Wrecking Ball (House Piano Extended) – Kar Play

Faded – Zhu

Bluebird Wine – Emmylou Harris and Rodney Crowell

Take Me to Church – Hozier

Latch – Disclosure featuring Sam Smith

Timebomb – Kylie Minogue

SexyBack – Justin Timberlake

Run-Around – Blues Traveler

Ooh La La – Goldfrapp

Come with Me Now – Kongos

Day 348, March 12, 2015

> *"Out of the woods by choice."*
> —Mumford & Sons, "Hopeless Wanderer"

I'm far from a world traveler, but it's hard not to notice how different one airport is from another.

In Kingston, for example, where I'm about to board my flight home via Atlanta, you wait in the shopping concourse until you hear your flight being called before you're permitted to approach departure gates.

It's a little like Penn Station in NYC, where hundreds of people line up single file to step on an escalator to get to their track.

So many things to worry about here, a. if you're a shopper (I am), and b. the queue for the escalator to the gates is very, very long. I remember paying for a daily pass to use the VIP lounge at the Montego Bay airport, which gets you directly to your gate when your flight is ready to board.

It didn't occur to me to do that in Kingston, and I'm concentrating on the (super quiet) boarding announcements so I'll make my flight.

Last night I felt a sense of unusual calm about my race on Saturday. It was not a moment too soon, because more than a few people around me have either (1) seemed exasperated with me or (2) told me straight out to let it go.

So okay, I'm trusting my training. The forecast is 100 percent rain, but I've already run in a (bitter cold)downpour. I haven't run long in three weeks, but I'm trusting my training and counting on fresh legs to get me to the finish.

You get the picture.

Yet fashion is on my mind. And color. As I'm usually in black, gray, navy, or white, one of the things I love about the running culture is the awesome pop of color, especially unnatural pink, yellow, and green. I'm not planning to drive downtown and won't have my car to stash anything, so I'll need some pockets for gummy bears and Swedish Fish, and my house key.

I'm hydrating like crazy so I don't need to tank up on Saturday, and I'm focusing on easy carbs.

🎵 PLAYLIST HIGHLIGHTS

My Rock 'n' Roll Playlist:

Here's what distance runner and fellow Kingston business traveler Patrick Gatti encouraged me to add.

Drops of Jupiter – Train

Can't Hold Us – Macklemore & Ryan Lewis

Raise Your Glass – Pink

And since I'm in Kingston, I've included this:

Who Knows – Protoje

Day 354, March 18, 2015

"Because I'm happy."
—Pharrell Williams, "Happy"

Here's what I know now.

It's always been 100 percent mental.

My first half marathon on Saturday was simply *clutch*.

Although I had put in the mileage a few weeks ago, I was coping with a lingering image of my skeleton crumbling at the start. This is a recurring nightmarish visual for me, and it takes enormous focus and brainpower to allow the more positive voices in my head to take over.

Triathlete drove me to 14th and Constitution Avenue while it was still dark, cold, and rainy. It was my idea to make a pit stop at the W Hotel a few blocks from the start. The hotel staff had set up coffee, juice, and fruit for runners, and there were plenty of us warming up on the black and white marble floors. I was well-rested and felt grateful for the support of random strangers and the good wishes from Mia, Adin, Lord Baltimore (who was in Africa), family, friends, and co-workers, as well as Really Smart, Buff, and Adorable.

Earlier in the week while I was working in Kingston, I had taken a look at the race route but then snapped my laptop shut when I caught a glimpse of the first big hill. In the car on Saturday morning, Triathlete asked me if I'd studied the route as she had suggested.

"No."

"Well, I did," she said. "That big hill you're worried about is at the six-mile mark, and since it's my neighborhood, I'll meet you there. Plan to walk up the hill to Calvert Street and use the break to have some of your Swedish Fish."

By the time I reached the hill, I had already taken a bathroom break at one of the Porta Potties (which were practically everywhere throughout the race route, although nearly all of them had long lines). I walked up the hill, ate my Swedish Fish, and chatted with her for a second or two. It was a nice break.

I continued along Calvert Street over to Mount Pleasant and Adams Morgan. I had passed the halfway mark and was feeling fine.

Absolutely fine.

Now the rain was pounding. My North Face jacket was soaked, and water was pooling in my cap. I made two more bathroom stops as I was hydrating every few miles and walked two more steep hills before crossing the finish line, which came sooner than I expected. My overall time was 3:16:38, much longer than I had planned, but I knew the lines at the bathrooms would mess with my race time.

I was thinking along the way that my goals for my next half marathon are to (1) minimize bathroom stops and (2) run up at least one steep hill.

***

You can build endurance and strengthen your muscles, but it's your brain that allows you to develop a strategy to get results in spite of the physical obstacles we all face at some point.

And since those obstacles tend to stack up on top of each other, you need to think through how you're going to remove them one by one if you want to see results.

For example, this time last year I avoided any exercise that might not be good for my left knee, which I had neglected to rehabilitate after surgery. No lunges, no squats, no running. I'm still not doing lunges or squats, because even though I know how good they are for strengthening my glutes, I get bone-on-bone contact that is like chalk on a blackboard.

So instead I strengthen my quads and the muscles around my knees, with the idea that these muscles will stabilize my knees. I use the recumbent bike as often as I can.

And for a year I've been doing straight-leg raises before bedtime, even if I'm actually in bed if I have to, after my other PT exercises. I think these have made all the difference in terms of stabilizing my knees, which by the way are just fine and always have been.

And that's just one example among many.

Although I can't control everything (I know, really), I'm careful about my form when I'm exercising because the possibility of twisting or otherwise injuring my knees freaks me out.

And of course, I'm swimming two or three days/week for 30 to 45 minutes depending on my schedule. I've noticed swimming strengthens my calves in addition to widening my aerobic window.

What's key about swimming, though, is that it's something I can do when I am otherwise suffering from a sore or tweaked muscle or even an injury. My goal is at least 1,500 yards, which is what *Runner's World* recommends for long-distance runners who are cross-training.

All of this is what my brain is telling me even as my body wants to sleep in or settle in with a glass of wine after work.

It has always been mental.

And I've learned to ask for help and support when I need it and how to know when I need it. I think this is one of the hardest things for many women (e.g., me), as we are all about being in control.

Throughout the past year I've felt more stupid more times than at any other point in my life. Yet I've forced myself to reach out (a lot) to all kinds of people around me for guidance and support.

I'm not an athlete, and I've never been one. Let's just say my Jewish upbringing was risk-averse.

"I'm glad you're okay," my father wrote me after the race.

Through it all, here is what my brain is telling me: I (still) want results.

- ◊ Weight loss
- ◊ Toned muscles
- ◊ A fit body
- ◊ Health and well-being

During a tough long run a few months ago with my running group, when I was clearly struggling at around mile 9, the coach stopped short.

"I need to have a pep talk with Carolee," she snapped.

Coach Lisa looked me in the eye.

"You're almost there."

It was the whole package. The group support, Lisa's words, her confidence.

Coach Lisa was right.

I am almost there.

Day 365, March 29, 2015

> *"I just hit my stride now."*
> —Emmylou Harris, "Bluebird Wine"

In the world of fitness journeys, I think Day 365 is probably a mega day.

It is in mine.

I haven't watched the *Biggest Loser* recently, but I love that show. It highlights how hard it is to change your lifestyle so you can simply feel good and be healthy. So much sustained effort and commitment is necessary, no matter how much you have to lose.

That's what's clutch. Whatever it is you want to accomplish is the only thing that is important.

I have a friend who has been running his entire adult life. He doesn't know how far he runs or how fast, but he's out the door five days a week. His goal each day?

"So I can run tomorrow."

For me, I set out to lose weight, strengthen and get lean, and be able to walk five blocks without running out of air.

It sounds simple, but if you've ever tried to shape up, you know how not simple all of this is. While I'm not where I want to be, I'm good with how far I've come.

And I'm having fun. I told Lord Baltimore over the weekend that I enjoy working out so much, I could exercise for six hours a day. If you want to invite me out for a run or to work out and then maybe go out for a drink, I will always say yes.

From Day 1, I was never 100 percent confident I would see change. But as I surrounded myself with experts I trusted and friends and family who didn't completely tune me out,

I did think this might work. Remember, I've never been looking for just a little change.

This journey is about RESULTS.

Early on I was having drinks with Ripped when I wondered aloud whether it was physically possible for me to kill the flab under my arms. Or on my stomach. Could just be the way I'm built.

Ripped didn't have an answer, and we were both quiet, thinking the same thing for half a second.

Yeah, that would suck.

It has not been a sprint since that conversation. Yet now when I text Mia and Adin with my run stats or race results, instead of "awesome" or "way to go," at least one of them, usually Mia, will comment on my outfit.

It's kind of breezy that neither one is surprised or even shocked that I'm moving around. They're almost *yeah whatever* when I've packed in eight miles between Bethesda and Georgetown on a random Sunday.

So, running. I never planned to be a runner, and running was never a goal. And I did not always enjoy running, either. It was my cousin Stephen Newman who told me if I could just push myself to get to three miles, the rest would be a piece of cake. Not exactly a piece of cake, but he was right. I don't know if that's how long it takes for endorphins to kick in, but by the time I hit three I am in a groove.

But I don't want to understate how freakin' hard it was to get to three. If you've been there, you know how crushing hard this is.

Where there have been challenges, there have also been some easy moments. For example, I've been digging the whole running fashion thing from Day 1. The colors, the amazing fabrics, the activewear vibe. From having been a person who'd never owned a single pair of sneakers 13 months ago, I am the one you want to talk to about stability versus neutral fit.

So fun.

It would be ridiculous not to say that the finish is my favorite part of a race. But now that I've done a few (10K Turkey Chase, 5.5K Sagicor run in Kingston, D.C. Rock 'n' Roll Half Marathon, and Sunday's 10K Alumrun), what I can admit to enjoying most is the warm-up.

That part where a DJ blasts "SexyBack" or "Fancy." You know what I'm talking about. Someone gets on a stage to lead the crowd in brisk exercises and dance moves. The best warm-up by far was in Kingston. No surprise there, and combined with the temperature in the low 80s and the bright sunshine, I kept thinking, *it doesn't get any better than this.*

I was surprised there was very little official warm-up at the D.C. Rock 'n' Roll Half Marathon. I was waiting so long for my corral to get a gun start, I plugged into my music and pumped it up. Okay, I got some looks, but mostly they were smiles (or chuckles).

Adorable told me before my first race to expect a party atmosphere. Those were his exact words. But when you think about it, even if you're expecting a party atmosphere, it's still *unexpected*. There is the potential at every passing mile of physical torture, so basically it would be like a torture party.

Every runner has got something going on in their head just before a race that's crazy private, but that's the community we share. We've all got our stories. I love looking around during the warm-up and wondering about that spark. We're all so different yet doing the same thing. How nuts is that?

And it's never been about the race part of the run, because I've never cared about my time or the competition.

My goal has always been calorie burn and pushing myself physically and mentally.

To that end I'm focusing on maintaining my form, keeping my breathing steady, paying attention to the trail around me, letting my mind visit places or discover creative ideas, and getting to the Finish.

But on the way to dinner at Summer House at the new Pike and Rose in Bethesda Sunday night, I logged on to Alumrun to check my finish time, and there it was.

1. Carolee Walker

First place in my gender/age category.

OMG.

I could seriously turn out to be that person who cares about her time.

I could be that person who passes up a bathroom break to get a better time and just lets it go.

I could be that runner who, instead of slowing down to take the cup of water from a volunteer's hand and pausing to say thank you, grabs the cup, takes a sip, and whips the cup and the rest of the water to the side of the road.

I know it's disgusting to pee on yourself, but apparently, it's what runners do (I hear) who care about their time.

(I'm envisioning high-powered water guns at the finish. Has anyone marketed these for runners?)

Random musings on Day 365:

Gear: I carry a lacrosse ball with me so I can massage the arches of my feet. If you're like me and still wearing heels to work, you have to keep up with this. Otherwise I've got pain on the bottom of my feet when I run that refuses to ease up no matter how cushy my Brooks are or how long I can balance on one foot with my eyes closed. If I can manage it, I'm also rolling my calves with either the lacrosse ball or a regular roller, which I do not have in my office (yet).

Food: I've become an attuned eater, always looking to fill my plate with what I need. I read in a fitness blog that one way to lose weight is to eat after a workout as if you haven't exercised. I understand what the writer was getting at, but I don't agree. You should be extremely deliberate about what you eat after you exercise. For example, in the evening after the 10k on Sunday at Summer House, I had a Blinker cocktail, substituting vodka for rye and shaken with pomegranate and grapefruit juice, calamari, and spicy tuna nigiri. Just what I needed.

Here's the greatest salad of all time, which I discovered in Kingston. I was eating it at the embassy one day, and a colleague asked me where I got it from. When I told him how much it cost (a lot), he was not deterred.

"Fifteen dollars of wonderfulness," he said.

If you need the extra protein, you can add grilled chicken or shrimp.

THE PERFECT (KINGSTON) SALAD

Ingredients

Handfuls of greens—any kind—with sprinklings of pea shoots or sunflower micro greens. I've used kale, but delicate greens are better.

¼ cup chickpeas (from a can, rinsed)

¼ cup black beans (from a can, rinsed)

¼ cup dried cranberries

¼ cup walnuts

Tiny bit of homemade mustard dressing or a homemade lemony vinaigrette

Instructions

Mix ingredients in a large bowl and serve.

Hydration: After my interview with the awesome Orioles nutritionist Sue James for an article I was writing, I now have a daily hydration plan. I've got to take in at least 74 ounces of water, and depending on how much driving I'm doing or what kind of meetings I'm attending, I need to have a plan.

Walking: Since coming back from Jamaica, when the weather has not been impossible, I am walking to all the places I regularly drive to. Dinner in Bethesda? Walk there. Farmer's market? Walk there. Even if I don't have any place to go, I am taking an evening walk or a lunchtime walk. My goal is two to three miles, but even if it's one mile because it's cold out or late, I'm getting in a walk.

I've finally managed the coordination to read or watch a movie while walking on the treadmill. So if I can't get outside, I'm catching up on book club reading and Netflix. I'm even thinking of putting a simple treadmill on next year's Chanukah list.

Whether or not it's a training day or a run day or a swim day, or even my workout day off, I'm walking. It's now a part of my day, like eating, sleeping, and brushing my teeth.

Supplements: Protein powder. I am having such positive results from the combination of whey powder and casein powder. I don't always take both on the same day, but on the day of a long run, I might. Sometimes I mix a scoop of whey powder with eight ounces of water just before training, which usually includes weights, and maybe just after depending on whether I have time to make an egg. I use the casein powder (one scoop with eight ounces of water) as dessert after dinner every other day. I bought the casein powder on Amazon because I couldn't find one locally that was not artificially sweetened. There are a few natural products out there, and they're easy to get online. Just don't be surprised that the container is practically the size of a large outdoor flowerpot.

Training: I am completely sold on this. At this point, 90 percent of what I do with Buff, I could not do on my own. My friend Chris noted that Adorable had the hard job of setting me up for success. He says Buff's got it easy now that I've got such great habits. Hmm. Here's what I think about training. If you can manage it, get yourself a trainer, if for no other reason than that your trainer is the exact person with whom to talk through your fitness goals.

No joke. If I can do this, so can you.

🎵 PLAYLIST HIGHLIGHTS

My Long Run Mix:

Incorporating some house.

No You Girls – Franz Ferdinand

Who Knows – Protoje

Walk Away – Jasmine V

Uptown Funk – Mark Ronson featuring Bruno Mars

Lighters – Bad Meets Evil featuring Bruno Mars

Come With Me Now – Kongos (Just so great.)

Time of Our Lives – Pitbull

Welcome to New York – Taylor Swift

Wrecking Ball – Kar Play

Faded – Zhu

Take Me To Church – Hozier

Love Hurts – Gram Parsons and Emmylou Harris

Latch – Disclosure featuring Sam Smith

Go Do – Jonsi

Got 2 Luv U – Sean Paul

Timebomb – Kylie Minogue

Dog Days Are Over – Florence + the Machine

The Con – Tegan and Sara

Closer to the Sun – Slightly Stoopid

Time after Time – Cyndi Lauper

Liquid Lunch – Caro Emerald

Summer – Calvin Harris

Right Round – Flo Rida

Run-Around – Blues Traveler

Mozart's House – Clean Bandit

We Run the Night – Havana Brown

212 – Azealia Banks

We Are the One – Pitbull

Comme Un Enfant – Yelle

Timber – Pitbull

Ooh La La – Goldfrapp

Club Can't Handle Me – Flo Rida

Rhythm of Love – Plain White Ts

Paper Planes – MIA

Switch – Will Smith

Fancy – Iggy Azalea

Wild Motion (Set It Free) – Miami Horror

Waiting Here (filous remix) – Jake Isaac

Cheap Sunglasses – RAC

Thunder Clatter – Wild Cub

Valerie – Amy Winehouse

The Wire – HAIM

Day 379, April 12, 2015

> *"You girls never know."*
> —Franz Ferdinand, "No You Girls"

As I'm setting new fitness goals, I can't get *Lean In* out of my head. I've spent the better part of my adult life holding myself back physically.

Most of the time, at the end of a long day, or any day, as well as on the weekends, I was looking to fill my time gently. I was seeking comfort. Movies, theater, spa treatments, books, sleep. Go to the gym? Are you kidding me? I biked a little, but I've always had a bike with a lot of gears, and you know which chain I locked into.

The one slight exception was skiing, which I learned to do at a young age. Growing up on the East Coast, I skied in subzero temperatures and icy conditions. But when I discovered Colorado and Utah, I became a vacation skier. Even now you won't catch me out there in bad weather. Powder, sunshine, barbeque lunches on the side of the mountain with California Coolers (do they still make these?).

A few years ago, it took a European ski instructor to trick me into learning how to ski the bumps. It was more like a hostage situation than a ski lesson.

When the small group of us, mostly men, got off the gondola, it looked like we had landed on the moon.

"What was it about *I don't ski bumps* that you did not get?" I asked René, I think his name was.

"If you don't learn to ski the bumps, there will always be too many."

Yeah, right.

"If you learn to ski the bumps, there will never be enough."

OMG, give me a break. I looked around at the group (guys), and it was like a frat party. They were practically giddy.

It wasn't that I was afraid to ski the bumps.

Okay, I was.

But I also thought it was stupid.

Like it's not enough to be at 6,000 feet above sea level with little minks darting in and out of aspens. We have to fabricate mounds of snow packed together two feet apart from each other creating an obstacle course as you head down the narrow slope of a mountain that looks like the edge of a skyscraper.

Stupid.

And annoying.

I thought all I needed to do was somehow get myself to the bottom and then do my own thing.

But I let René teach me how to ski the fucking bumps.